Atlas of Ophthalmology

Presented as a Service to Ophthalmic Medicine by Fisons plc manufacturers of

Opticrom®

Sodium Cromoglycate BP

Further product information is available from Fisons plc Pharmaceutical Division 12 Derby Road, Loughborough Leicestershire LE11 0BB

ATLAS OF OPHTHALMOLOGY

Michael G. Glasspool, FRCS, DO

Consultant Ophthalmologist,
Orpington Hospital and Queen Mary's Hospital, Sidcup, Kent

Published, in association with
UPDATE PUBLICATIONS LTD., by

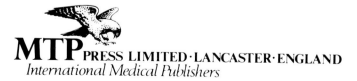

MTP PRESS LIMITED · LANCASTER · ENGLAND
International Medical Publishers

Published, in association with
Update Publications Ltd, by

MTP Press Limited
Falcon House
Lancaster, England

Reprinted 1984

British Library Cataloguing in Publication Data

Glasspool, Michael G.
    Atlas of ophthalmology.
    1. Ophthalmology
    I. Title
    617.7   RE 46

    ISBN 0-85200-434-6

Printed by Cradley Print PLC,
Cradley Heath, Warley, W. Midlands

Contents

Preface

This book is designed to be a pictorial guide to ophthalmology and not a comprehensive textbook.

It includes chapters on anatomy, physiology and optics to explain the simple elements of the basic sciences that are needed to understand ophthalmology.

The section on examination describes the common investigations in an eye department in the hope that reports from ophthalmologists may become more easily understood.

The clinical chapters represent 5 years of ophthalmic referrals by local family doctors in a part rural and part suburban area. This selection of eye disease therefore excludes some of the rare conditions, but includes those common problems that can worry not only the busy family doctor, but also the hard pressed medical student.

Anatomy and Physiology

1

The sense of vision depends on the integrity of a set of anatomical and physiological factors, a study of which will simplify the understanding of ocular disease.

External Eye

The eyeball lies in the anterior part of the orbit, which is approximately pyramidal in shape. The bony orbital margin, which outlines the base of the pyramid, affords some protection to the globe from blunt injury. The close relationship of the orbit to the frontal, maxillary, ethmoidal and sphenoidal sinuses can be of great importance when these structures are diseased.

The exposed portion of the eye is covered by the upper and lower lids. These distribute not only the tear film over the cornea but also the oily secretion from the Meibomian glands, which slows the evaporation of the tear film. The Meibomian glands are modified sebaceous glands situated within the tarsal plate—a fibrous reinforcement of the lids. The lids join at the medial and lateral canthus. At the medial canthus is the fleshy caruncle with the plica semilunaris—a vestigial nictitating membrane (Figure 1).

The lacrimal gland lies behind the outer third of the upper lid. Tears enter the conjunctival sac in the upper fornix—a cul-de-sac which prevents contact lenses from disappearing behind the eye! The drainage of tears takes place via the upper and lower puncta at the medial ends of the lids. Thence the lacrimal canaliculi join to enter the lacrimal sac which lies nasal to the medial canthus.

The nasolacrimal duct connecting the sac to the inferior meatus of the nose is a common site for obstruction, resulting in a watering eye (epiphora) in the new-born (Figure 2).

Internal Eye

The eye consists of three concentric layers. The outermost fibrous sclera is opaque and accounts for five sixths of the globe. It is continued anteriorly into the transparent cornea. The middle vascular coat or uveal tract is made up of the choroid, ciliary body and iris. The innermost layer is the light sensitive retina formed embryologically from the forebrain vesicle (Figure 3).

The corneal epithelium is continuous with the conjunctiva covering the sclera and lining the lids. Defects in this layer are very painful because of its rich nerve supply, but heal rapidly without scarring. Damage to the deeper layers results in permanent changes and the loss of normal transparency. The corneal endothelium is

Figure 1. *External eye.*

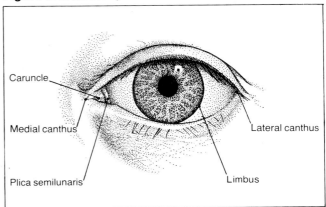

Caruncle

Medial canthus

Lateral canthus

Plica semilunaris

Limbus

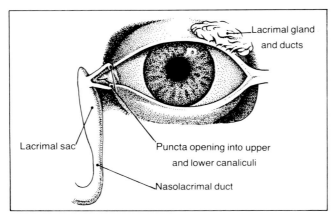

Figure 2. *Lacrimal system.*

Figure 3. *Horizontal cross-section of the eye.*

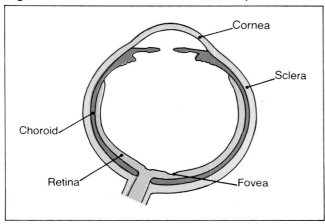

Figure 4. *The anterior segment of the eye.*

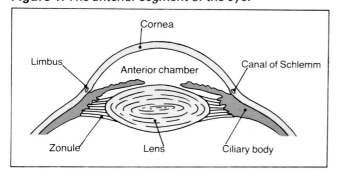

vital to the maintenance of corneal clarity as damage allows water to enter the stroma causing a ground glass appearance. This disruption is the cause of the bullous keratopathy seen after cataract extraction. The normal absence of blood vessels in the cornea is the reason for the high success rate of corneal grafts.

The anterior chamber is bounded by the cornea in front and the iris behind. In the small hypermetropic eye the depth of the chamber may be shallow and thus predispose to acute glaucoma, but in myopia the eye is longer and the angle between the iris and cornea is wide open.

The lens lies behind the iris within a capsule which is attached to the muscle of the ciliary body by a series of fine fibres—the zonule.

Aqueous humour is secreted by the epithelium of the ciliary body and passes forward through the pupil. It leaves the eye after passing through a fine sieve (trabecular meshwork) overlying the canal of Schlemm, which encircles the eye at the junction of the cornea and sclera—the limbus (Figure 4).

The vitreous humour is the transparent medium which fills the eye behind the lens. It consists of a three-dimensional scaffold of collagen fibres and hyaluronic acid. With degeneration of the vitreous the fibres come to lie together and are seen by the patient as 'floaters'. Stimulation of the retina can occur by traction of the vitreous and the patient may then see flashes of light or sparks. These symptoms frequently occur in the early stages of retinal detachment when a tear is developing in the retina.

The light-sensitive cells of the retina are rods and cones—so called because of their shape. They lie in the outer layer in contact with the pigment epithelium which is vital for their metabolism. Various conditions of the retina may cause dispersion of the pigment such that inflammation produces black clumps, and retinitis pigmentosa is associated with a typical bone-corpuscle formation.

Mechanism of Vision

The visual pigments in the rods and cones initiate the transformation of light into a series of electrical impulses for transmission to the visual cortex in the occipital lobes. Each pigment absorbs light from a different part of the visible spectrum (Figure 5). The pigment in rods is rhodopsin and absorbs blue-green light. Each cone contains one of three pigments for the blue, green and yellow wavelengths.

The cones are responsible for photopic vision and respond to bright light and colours, while the rods mediate scotopic vision and react to low levels of illumination, but do not distinguish colours. Therefore in daylight it is principally the cones which function while in moonlight it is the rods that are active. After a period in poor light the process of dark adaptation increases the sensitivity of the rods to produce 'night

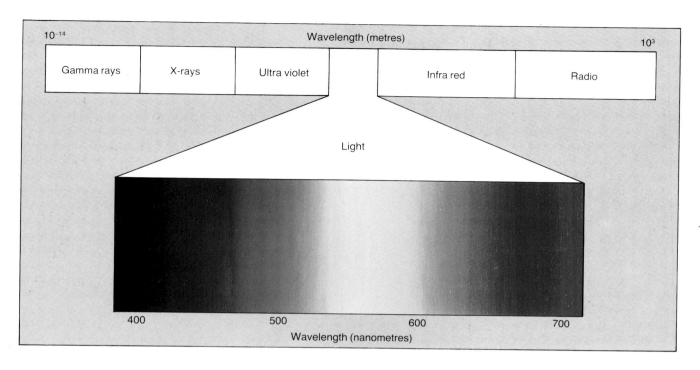

Figure 5. *Spectrum of electromagnetic radiation.*

vision'. As the rods are concentrated away from the macula the peripheral vision is better than the central vision. This explains why it is easier to see a star at night by looking to one side of it.

Colour vision is achieved by cone pigments and a deficiency or absence of any of these pigments produces colour blindness. As colour blindness is genetically determined on a sex-linked recessive basis it is commoner amongst men, the incidence being about eight per cent for men and 0.4 per cent for women.

The electrical changes that occur in the retina when it is stimulated by a flash of light can be recorded by means of a corneal electrode embedded in a contact lens and another applied to the forehead. The action potential, or electroretinogram (ERG), depends on the normal state of the various retinal layers. It may be used clinically to explain defective vision in childhood or in the early diagnosis of inherited retinal degeneration, such as retinitis pigmentosa, when the fundus may appear normal. It is also possible to record occipital cortex activity by means of scalp electrodes. This visually evoked response (VER) reflects the function of the fovea and central visual pathways and may be combined with an electroencephalogram (EEG) where other brain damage is suspected. The nerve fibres in the retina run towards the optic disc on the temporal side in an arching fashion as they are displaced by the bulk of the macular fibres. Lesions of the optic disc (glaucoma,

vascular occlusions) therefore give arcuate field defects.

The fibres pass in the optic nerve to meet and partially mix at the optic chiasma. The nasal fibres from each eye cross to the opposite side, while the temporal fibres do not cross.

From the chiasma the pathway is via the optic tracts to the lateral geniculate bodies where the fibres synapse. The optic radiation passes around the lateral ventricle to the visual cortex of the occipital lobe.

The site of any lesion producing a visual field defect can be localized by reference to this anatomical pathway (Figure 6).

Muscles of the Eye

Each eye is moved by four rectus muscles (superior, inferior, medial and lateral) and two oblique muscles (superior and inferior).

The insertions on the eye of these muscles are such that they have a main action and secondary actions. Only the medial and lateral recti move the eye in a simple horizontal direction. From Figure 7 it is possible to see that the superior rectus elevates the eye and has a secondary action of adducting and intorting the eye. Torsion of the eye occurs about an anteroposterior axis. While the superior rectus is contracting, the opposite inferior oblique (contralateral synergist) will move the other eye in the same direction.

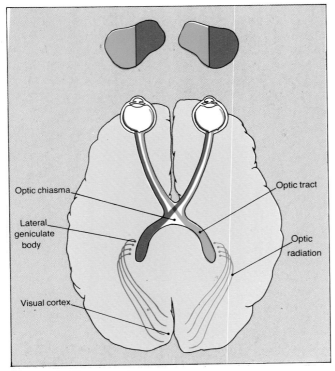

Figure 6. *Nerve pathways.*

Figure 7. *Actions of eye muscles.*

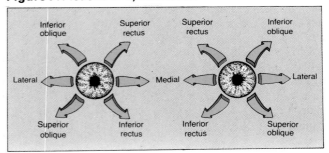

Binocular single vision is achieved by the fusion of the two retinal images by the brain. This depends on a sharply defined image from each eye, normal muscular co-ordination and the ability of the brain to fuse the two pictures.

The advantages include an enlarged visual field and three-dimensional vision with, in addition, improved visual acuity and compensation for the blind spot of each eye by the other.

Normal binocular vision is acquired by the age of three years, but alterations in vision can occur up to the age of seven or eight years. For this reason it is imperative to correct squints early, to prevent amblyopia or lazy eye.   □

Examination of the Eye

2

Management of eye disease causes considerable anxiety for most doctors. However, the eye is unique in offering an opportunity for relatively easy assessment and early diagnosis of not only local ocular conditions, but also many systemic diseases, the identification of which would otherwise require complicated, expensive and time-consuming investigations.

Visual Acuity

Distance vision is assessed with a Snellen Chart set at 6 m from the patient or at 3 m when viewed through a mirror. Each of the patient's eyes is tested separately, with the patient covering the other eye with a piece of card. Vision is recorded from 6/60 (the top letter) to a normal 6/6, although 6/5 or 6/4 can be read by some (Figure 1).

If the vision is below normal the chart should be viewed through a 1 or 2 mm hole punched in a piece of card (this can be easily done with the tip of a ball-point pen). If the visual acuity improves then a refractive error is present and a test for glasses is necessary. If there is no improvement, further ocular examination is indicated.

When the top letter cannot be read, the patient is asked to try and count the examiner's fingers (CF) or failing this, to assess hand movements (HM). The minimum vision recorded is perception of light (PL).

Near vision is recorded from N.5, the smallest, to N.24 (Figure 2).

Visual Fields

Accurate charting of peripheral and central fields requires equipment that is usually found only in eye clinics.

Peripheral fields are assessed on a self-recording perimeter, in which either a test target or a test stimulus from a projected light is moved along an arc, of radius one third of a metre rotatable for exploration of every meridian (Figure 3).

Central fields can be charted using a Bjerrum screen. This method is used to investigate the area of the visual field extending to include the blind spot (Figure 4). When extreme accuracy is required, combined peripheral and central fields may be examined with a projection perimeter. The test stimulus, which can be adjusted for size, intensity and colour is projected on to the inner surface of a constant and uniformly illuminated hemisphere (Figure 5).

Semi-automatic visual field analysers are also used by opticians. These present a random series of stimuli to the patient. The test is rapid and can be conducted by unskilled technicians.

For a quick, easy assessment requiring no complicated equipment the confrontation method can be used. The doctor and patient each cover opposite eyes and fix each other's uncovered eye. Using a hat pin or the fingers, a comparison is made between the visual field of the patient and that of the examiner. A check can be kept on the fixation of the patient (Figure 6).

An estimate of central defects can be gauged if the patient is asked to count the fingers of the examiner's hands in the four quadrants of the visual field.

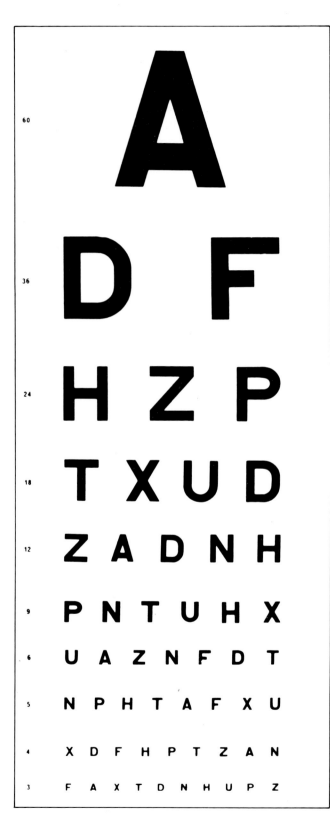

Figure 1. *A Snellen chart, which must be 6 m from the patient.*

Colour Vision

Several methods are available to assess colour vision, but the so-called Ishihara plates are most commonly used. These comprise a series of pseudo-isochromatic cards. The normal person can read all the letters or figures but someone with defective colour vision is unable to do so. The practical application lies in the detection of colour blindness in relation to different occupations. With the more sensitive methods it is also possible to detect early macular and optic nerve damage in toxic amblyopia and optic neuritis.

Intraocular Pressure

Intraocular pressure can be measured accurately only with the applanation tonometer (Figure 7). This requires a slit lamp and is a skilled technique. Non-contact tonometers are particularly popular amongst opticians as no local anaesthetic is required. However, the results can be very inaccurate. Digital tonometry is inaccurate for small rises in pressure (as in chronic simple glaucoma), but can be useful when the difference between the two eyes is marked as in acute glaucoma. The index fingers of each hand are used, with the other outstretched fingers resting on the forehead (Figure 8).

External Examination

Light and Magnification

Examination of the external eye must be carried out with good illumination and some form of magnification. A moveable desk light is best for general examination of the face and lids, but a torch or the light from an ophthalmoscope should be used for examining the eye ball. Magnification with a ×10 loupe (Figure 9) will show defects of the cornea and anterior chamber which are invisible to the naked eye. Because of the short focal length of the lens the examiner must be close to the patient.

Lids and Eyeball

The position of the lids in relation to each other and to the globe is noted, together with the degree of closure when the eyes are shut. The latter is of importance with VII nerve palsy or proptosis of the eyeball. No face is perfectly symmetrical and slight degrees of congenital asymmetry are common. Occasionally, this may give rise to a suspicion of some recent change, especially if there is apparent displacement of the eyeball. Old photographs of the patient may then help to date the deformity.

N.5

Such very small print as this is used only for special cases, for example, the small advertisements and financial columns in some magazines, for indexes and references, and pocket-sized bibles and prayerbooks.

ewers—save—seam—crease

N.6

This type size, the smallest in general use, is used in some newspapers for the classified advertisements, in telephone directories and timetables, and other such lists and reference books.

museum—cone—nave—sun

N.8

Most of the daily newspapers use this as the average size of print for their news columns. The letters are sometimes larger than this, but rarely are they smaller.

crown—serve—seen—newer

N.10

Magazines, novels and textbooks are usually set in characters of about this size, as are printed instructions.

ream—ear—venom—ruse

N.12

Books which are printed on very large pages, with many words on each line, often use a type similar to this one.

mane—sue—smear—sores

N.14

Titles of books and headings to paragraphs in newspapers are often set in type of this size, but usually in CAPITAL LETTERS.

mere—crane—oar—summer

N.18

BOLD headlines and children's books.

rose—one—scour—never

N.24

ADVERTISEMENTS, display.

Figure 2. *Near-vision test type. Letter size ranges from N.5 to N.24.*

Everting the Upper Lid

When a foreign body is suggested by the history, or there is a possibility of changes of the inside of the lid as in allergic conjunctivitis or trachoma, the upper lid must be everted. The patient is asked to look down and the upper lid lashes are firmly held. While the lashes are pulled slightly up and away from the globe, pressure is applied with a pen, glass rod or finger tip to the upper border of the tarsal plate (Figure 10). This lies about 1 cm away from the lid margin.

Cornea

The normal cornea has a bright reflex due to the tear film. If there is any deficiency in tear production (dry eye syndrome), this reflex is reduced and the normal tear strip along the lower lid margins is absent. The cornea is clear out to the limbus except when there is an arcus formation (this will be described later in the series). Superficial damage to the cornea from foreign bodies or abrasions is extremely painful. The use of a weak anaesthetic (minims benoxinate hydrochloride) will relieve the pain sufficiently to allow an adequate examination of the eye.

Fluorescein

Large corneal abrasions can often readily be seen with good illumination, but for identification of the smaller ones the application of fluorescein dye is necessary. The

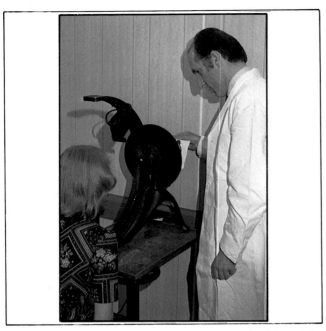

Figure 3. *Testing the peripheral field of vision. The patient watches a fixed central spot and states when the moving target becomes visible.*

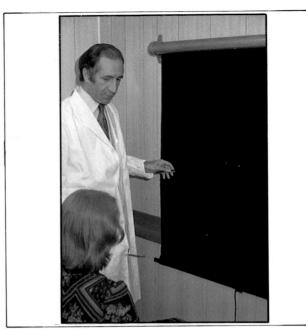

Figure 4. *Testing the central field of vision. This is determined by a method similar to that described in the caption to Figure 3.*

most convenient method is the use of fluorescein impregnated paper strips (Fluorets) (Figure 11), which are applied to the lower fornix. When the patients blinks, the dye is distributed over the cornea and conjunctiva, and stains any area where there is a break in the epithelium (Figure 12).

Internal Examination

Anterior Chamber

The depth of the anterior chamber must be assessed before the pupil is dilated. In the normal eye or in the myopic eye, the iris lies well back from the cornea and the angle between the iris and the cornea is about 45 degrees. The anterior chamber is shallow if the iris appears convex and seems to be lining the inside of the cornea.

The Pupil Reactions

The direct pupillary response is tested with the patient looking at the distance test chart. A brisk, maintained contraction of the pupil occurs when a bright torch or ophthalmoscope light is shone on the eye. The consensual reaction is the constriction of the contralateral pupil in response to light. The near reflex is elicited by

Figure 5. *Projection perimeter. This is the most sensitive estimation of central and peripheral fields. Note that the examiner can watch the patient through the telescope to check that the patient maintains her fixation.*

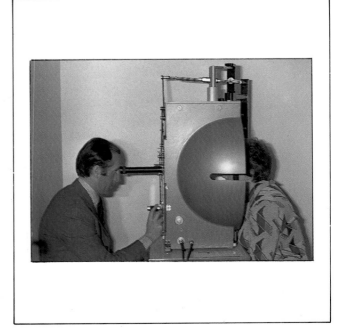

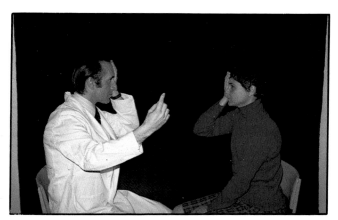

Figure 6. *Confrontation test. A simple test for peripheral field loss requiring no equipment.*

Figure 7. *Applanation tonometer. This is used to measure accurately the intraocular pressure (normally 15 to 20 mm Hg).*

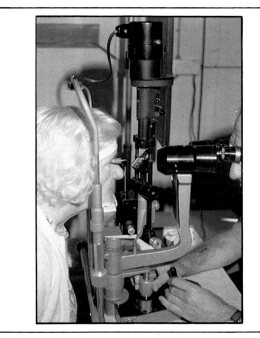

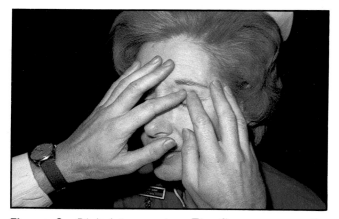

Figure 8. *Digital tonometry. The fingers assess the softness of each eye. This is an inaccurate method but is useful for acute glaucoma.*

Figure 9. *Loupe. A magnifying lens is necessary to see details of the front of the eye.*

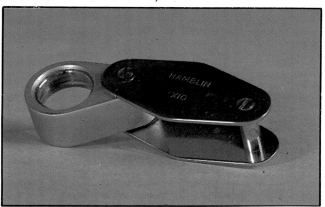

asking the patient to look into the distance and then to look suddenly at the examiner's finger held 10 cm from him. The constriction is less marked than that stimulated by light.

Ocular Movements

The examination for any deviation of the eyes is carried out by watching the corneal reflection of a torch or ophthalmoscope light, which is held at a distance of 30 cm. Normally, the reflection in each eye is slightly nasal to the centre of the cornea. If the eye is convergent the reflection is displaced temporally, while in the divergent eye the light reflex is seen nearer the limbus on the nasal side.

Smaller deviations may need the cover test to show up the defect. This will be described in the article on 'Squints'.

Mobility of each eye is tested with one eye covered, while the other eye follows the light as it is moved in all directions of gaze. Defects identified by this test, such as an inability to abduct one eye with a VI nerve palsy, may help to point to an affected muscle (see action of muscles on page 11).

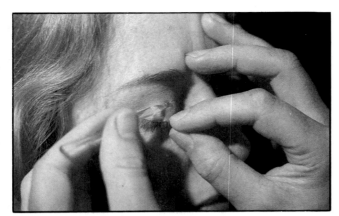

Figure 10. *Eversion of the upper lid. Counter-pressure is applied on the lid while the lashes are pulled upwards.*

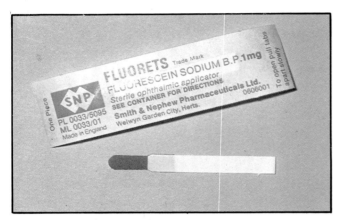

Figure 11. *Fluorescein. A convenient method for the application of the correct amount of dye from a sterile strip.*

Figure 12. *Application of fluorescein. The tip of a paper strip is wetted by the tears in the lower fornix.*

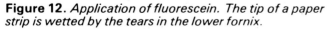

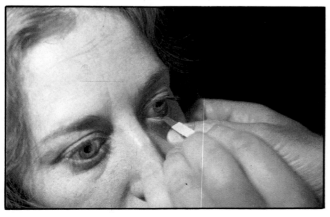

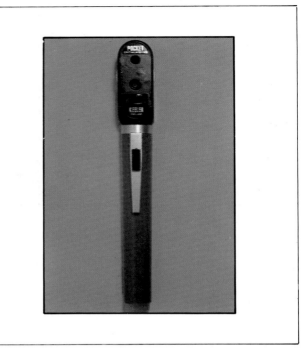

Figure 13. *General practitioners should have an ophthalmoscope as part of a diagnostic set.*

Symptoms may be related to a weakness of convergence, which is tested by asking the patient to look at the point of a pencil while it is gradually brought closer Normal convergence should enable the pencil to be brought to within 10 cm of the nose before the patient sees double.

Ophthalmoscopy

The ophthalmoscope is to the eye what the stethoscope is to the chest. There are many ophthalmoscopes available, but the Keeler Standard or Practitioner models which can be combined with an otoscope, are amongst the best (Figure 13). A pocket version may be preferred for convenience of size. All have the great advantage of the possibility of selection of different light beams. The narrow beam allows examination of the macula through an undilated pupil.

The examination begins with the ophthalmoscope set at 0, when no lenses are placed between the patient and examiner. If the examiner normally wears glasses, he may either continue to use them and dial 0, or take them off and adjust the ophthalmoscope lenses to the same power as that of his own glasses. If the patient is viewed from 30 cm the red reflex from the fundus is visible. The whole pupillary aperture is filled by an even red glow from light reflected from the choroidal vessels. Any

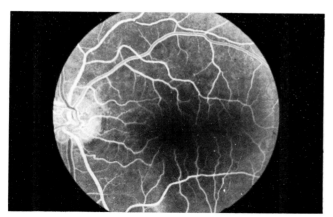

Figure 14. *Fluorescein angiography. Intravenous fluorescein outlining the retinal and choroidal circulation of the normal fundus.*

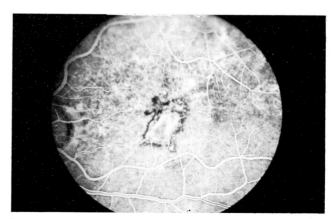

Figure 15. *Fluorescein angiography. Leakage of dye is seen in the region of the macula affected by disciform degeneration.*

opacities in the media, i.e. cornea, aqueous, lens or vitreous, will appear as a black silhouette against the red reflex.

If the examiner approaches the patient's eye, changes in the vitreous may become visible as dots, small wisps or swirling cobwebs. These characteristically change position as the eye moves.

Examination of the fundus should start at the disc, which lies slightly nasal to the macula. The patient is instructed to look straight ahead and the examiner approaches the eye from the temporal side, aiming at an imaginary point in the centre of the head. The disc should then be visible.

The peripheral retina is then viewed and the macular area left until last. This delays the intense pupillary constriction until the end of the examination.

In high myopia it is often easier to examine the fundus through the patient's glasses instead of trying to dial a high minus correction on the ophthalmoscope. In all cases the examiner's right eye is used for the patient's right eye and the left eye for the patient's left eye. If a clear view cannot be obtained it may be necessary to dilate the pupil. Mydriacyl (Alcon) is the ideal drug as it has a quick onset (10 minutes), it does not affect accommodation severely, and it wears off within six hours. On no account should homatropine or atropine be used because of the duration of their action.

Fluorescein Angiography

If fluorescein dye is injected intravenously it is possible to photograph its passage through the eye. The dye becomes bound to plasma albumin, to which the retinal vessels are impermeable. The normal appearance

Figure 16. *Ultrasonography. Horizontal B-scan section through a normal eye. (By courtesy of Miss M. Restori, Ultrasound Dept., Moorfields Eye Hospital.)*

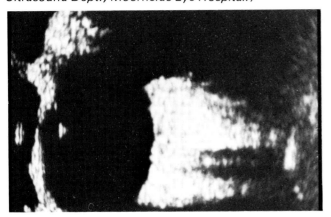

Figure 17. *Ultrasonography. Horizontal B-scan section through total retinal detachment with dense subretinal haemorrhage. (By courtesy of Miss M. Restori, Ultrasound Dept., Moorfields Eye Hospital.)*

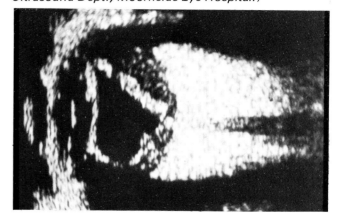

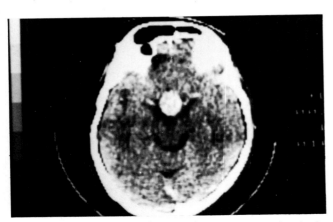

Figure 18. *EMI scan. Section at the level of the pituitary fossa showing a tumour which has been enhanced by dye. (By courtesy of The Neurosurgical Unit, Brook Hospital, London.)*

Figure 19. *Skull radiograph. Lateral view of patient in Figure 18 showing erosion of pituitary fossa.*

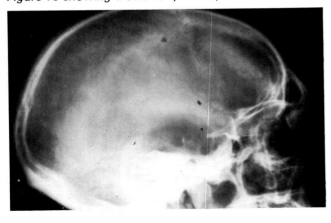

(Figure 14) shows the retinal vessels standing out against the fainter fluorescence from the choroidal vessels. When there is a defect in the retinal vessels or the pigment epithelium, leakage of the dye occurs (Figure 15).

This technique has helped in the diagnosis and treatment of many of the common vascular disorders of the retina.

Ultrasonography

When the ocular media are opaque and it is impossible to see the retina, ultrasonic examination can be used to assess the anatomy.

High frequency sound waves beamed at the eye produce echoes which can be converted into a picture on a cathode ray tube (Figure 16).

This technique can aid in the planning of possible surgery for vitreous haemorrhage or retinal detachment (Figure 17). It can also be used for investigation of the orbit and optic nerve abnormalities.

CT Scan

The EMI scanner system is a computer aided x-ray technique, the results of which can be shown on a cathode ray tube (Figure 18). The picture represents the image of a slice of tissue and considerable resolution of detail is possible (Figure 19). This non-invasive method has largely taken over the role of carotid angiography. □

PRACTICAL POINTS

Some ophthalmological examinations are easy to do in the surgery

* **Visual acuity — visual fields — colour vision**

* **External appearance — asymmetry, corneal abrasions, foreign bodies (evert upper lid)**

* **Internal appearance — anterior chamber, pupil reactions**

* **Eye movements**

* **Ophthalmoscopy — underused; develop a practised routine (see article text)**

* **Digital tonometry — inaccurate can mislead with chronic glaucoma**

For sophisticated techniques refer to ophthalmologist

* **Visual fields — detailed charts**

* **Applanation tonometry — the only accurate measurement**

* **Fluorescein angiography — i.v. injection; retinal vessels are shown well**

* **Ultrasonography — if retina is difficult to see**

* **CT scan — non-invasive; is now replacing carotid angiography**

Errors of Refraction and their Correction 3

Refraction

The term refraction is used by the physicist to describe the bending or deviation of a ray of light when it passes obliquely between two different media. If the medium through which it passes is a pane of glass with parallel sides, no deviation occurs, but if one side of the glass is curved the direction of the light is altered (Figure 1). In ophthalmology the term refraction is applied to the testing of the eyes for glasses.

Image Formation

The eye forms an image on the retina by focussing with the cornea and the lens, each of these acting as a convex lens.

The iris is the regulator of the amount of light reaching the retina, in the same way as the diaphragm regulates light entry into a camera. The retinal image is inverted so that the lower half of the retina sees the top half of an object, while the upper retina sees the lower part of the object. In this respect it is similar to a pinhole camera (Figure 2).

Accommodation

In the normal (emmetropic) eye, parallel rays are focussed on the retina when the ciliary muscle is relaxed (Figure 3).

If a near object is viewed, the process of accommo-

dation increases the power of the lens to produce a sharp retinal image (Figure 4).

Presbyopia

In childhood the power of accommodation is strong, so that objects can easily be seen only 10 cm away. With increasing age the power diminishes as a result of hardening and enlarging of the lens, so that glasses may be required for near work after the age of 45 years. This process is called presbyopia (Figure 5).

Figure 1. *Refraction of light.*

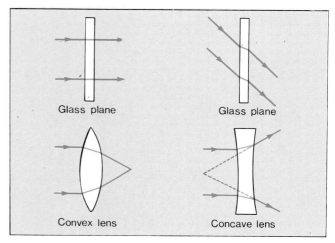

21

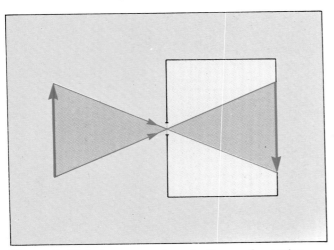

Figure 2. *Pinhole camera. Inverted image formation.*

Figure 3. *Parallel rays are focussed on the retina by the cornea and lens in the normal eye (emmetropia).*

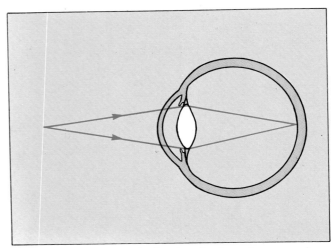

Figure 4. *Accommodation by the lens forms a sharp retinal image of a near object.*

Figure 5. *Presbyopia. Correction with a convex lens.*

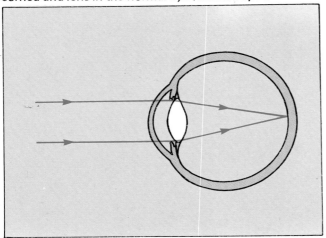

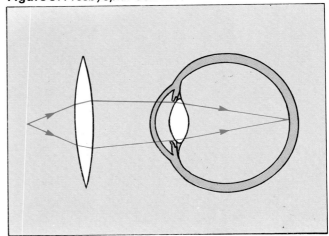

Errors of Refraction

Errors of refraction are of three kinds—myopia, hypermetropia and astigmatism—and are usually related to the shape and size of the eye (Figure 6).

Myopia

In myopia, or short sight, the eyeball is longer than normal so that the image of distant objects is formed in front of the retina (Figure 7). Any attempt to accommodate increases the blurring of the image, but near objects may be seen clearly (Figure 8). The distance vision can be corrected using a minus or concave lens (Figure 9).

In old age the process of nuclear sclerosis, or hardening of the lens, causes short sight so that the patient who previously required glasses for reading is able to do without them. This is unfortunately at the expense of the distance vision for which glasses become necessary.

Hypermetropia

In hypermetropia, or long sight, the eye ball is shorter than normal and the image in the resting eye is formed behind the retina. (Figure 10). The process of accommodation will compensate if the degree of hypermetropia is small, but with increasing age presbyopia limits the clarity of vision. This occurs first for near vision and later for distance vision. Therefore, reading

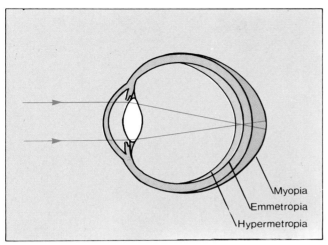

Figure 6. *Refractive errors. Hypermetropia, emmetropia, myopia.*

Figure 7. *Myopia. Blurred distance vision.*

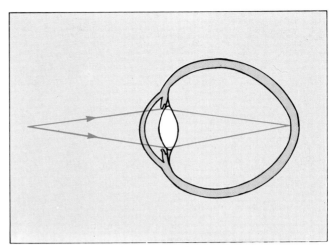

Figure 8. *Myopia. Clear near vision.*

Figure 9. *Myopia. Distance vision corrected with a concave lens.*

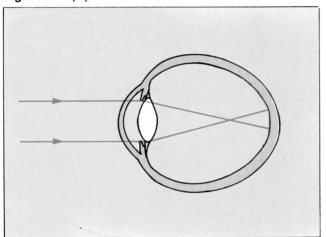

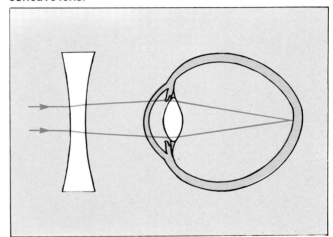

glasses may be needed by the age of 30 years and a distance correction soon afterwards (Figure 11).

After cataract extraction the eye is strongly hypermetropic. The correction of this error and its complications will be covered in the section on cataracts.

Astigmatism

In astigmatism there is unequal focussing of light in different meridians so that a sharp image cannot be achieved (Figure 12). A simple analogy can be made by comparing the lens system of the eye with the back of a spoon, when the long axis has a different curvature from that across the bowl. Nearly all eyes are affected to a greater or lesser extent by astigmatism. Attempts to correct the defect by accommodation are not successful and the use of cylindrical lenses is necessary (Figure 13).

Methods of Correcting Errors of Refraction

Glasses

The *dioptre* is the measurement of power of a lens. A convex lens of one dioptre power will bring parallel rays of light to a focus at 1 m (Figure 14).

Lenses for glasses are ground to the appropriate spherical power to correct hypermetropia or myopia. In addition, a cylindrical lens may be needed when there is astigmatism.

Usually the whole lens is used, but with high power prescriptions for myopia or after cataract extractions, a

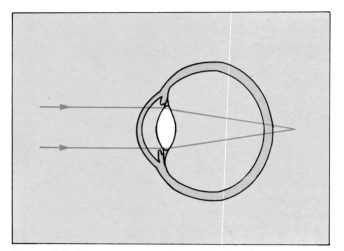

Figure 10. *Hypermetropia. Blurred vision for distance.*

Figure 11. *Hypermetropia. Correction with a convex lens.*

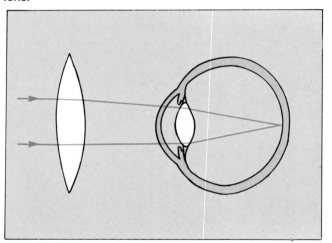

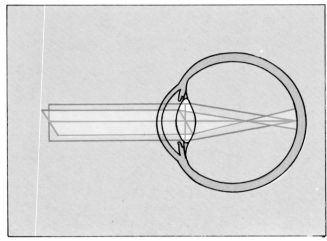

Figure 12. *Astigmatism. Blurred distance and near vision.*

Figure 13. *Astigmatism. Correction using cylindrical lens.*

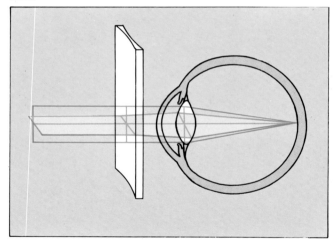

lenticular lens may be prescribed when only the centre portion is used for vision. The advantage is in reduced weight and thickness of the lens, but the cosmetic appearance is not always acceptable to the patient.

Bifocals are prescribed when a combination of distance and near lenses is required. Differing shapes of the reading segment are available depending on the patient's occupation. When there is difficulty in seeing clearly in the intermediate range, from 1 to 2 m, a variable focal lens can help. These lenses are made so that there is a steadily increasing power of the lower half of the lens. They have the disadvantage of some peripheral distortion when the patient looks down to the side, and they are expensive.

Tinting of lenses may be necessary if there is any degree of photophobia. A lens with a variable tint that changes with the amount of ultraviolet light is called a photochromatic lens.

Contact Lenses

There are three types of contact lenses: scleral, corneal and soft.

Scleral lenses made of hard plastic have a central optical area covering the cornea and a peripheral area which rests on the sclera. (Figure 15). Fitting these lenses involves taking a mould of the eye and many subsequent minor modifications. They are bulky and cannot be worn for long periods and are, therefore, rarely used.

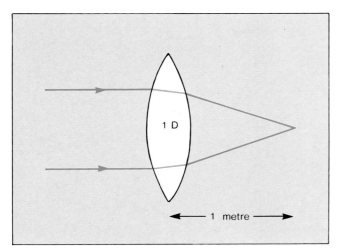

Figure 14. *The dioptre. Strength of a lens with a focal length of 1 m.*

Figure 15. *Scleral lens. Large plastic lens with the mould of the cornea.*

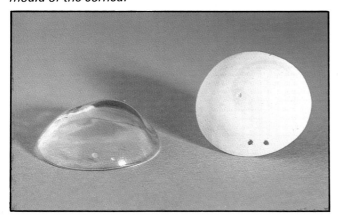

Corneal lenses have a diameter slightly smaller than that of the cornea and are also made in hard plastic. (Figure 16). They allow free flow of tears across the cornea and are well tolerated.

Soft lenses are made of soft plastic which can take up water like a sponge, and they are slightly larger than the corneal diameter (Figure 17). The softness of the lenses makes them extremely comfortable, but the vision is usually poorer than that achieved with a hard lens.

The presence of a contact lens on the cornea upsets the normal physiology by limiting the oxygen supply. This may be partially corrected in scleral lenses by drilling holes in the lens to allow a freer exchange of tears around the lens.

Corneal hypoxia does not occur with corneal lenses providing they are correctly fitted and worn. Because soft lenses contain water, these are the most physiological. Different makes of soft lenses have differing water uptake and, therefore, oxygen permeability. Those with 85 per cent water uptake can be worn continuously, but only under close supervision by an ophthalmologist.

Indications for Contact Lenses

Contact lenses may be needed for optical or practical reasons.

The optical indications are for the correction of myopia and hypermetropia. The distortions of high-power lenses for both these errors can be corrected with contact lenses. Often, both the visual acuity and the field of vision is improved. Generally, the higher the degree of the error the greater are the benefits.

Aphakia. When only one eye is affected by cataract, it is impossible to correct the vision after surgery with glasses. This is due to the increase by one third in the retinal image size in the affected eye. If a contact lens is worn the difference in the image size in each eye is negligible and the two eyes can work together.

Keratoconus. In this condition the cornea gradually becomes conical, producing marked astigmatism. This cannot be fully corrected by glasses, but is usually helped by contact lenses. The lenses do not delay the progress of the condition, but they may postpone the time when surgery is necessary.

The practical indications for contact lenses are for those patients who find that the wearing of glasses is incompatible with their activities. Included in this group are those who wear lenses for cosmetic reasons.

Contact lenses are generally used to correct distance vision only, so that reading glasses are also needed if the patient is presbyopic. Bifocal contact lenses are available but present too many difficulties to make their use widespread.

The general management of hard lenses is much easier than that of soft lenses. They are easier to keep clean without damage and their handling does not require the same meticulous care. Soft lens cleaning is a major drawback and must be either by heat pasteurization, which is tedious, or by chemicals, which has complications, mainly irritation of the eyes.

Complications of Contact Lenses

The over-wear syndrome is a common problem and is caused by a sudden increase in the time for which the lenses are worn. The patient awakes with very painful, watering eyes caused by damage to the corneal epi-

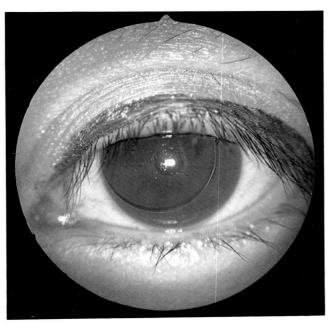

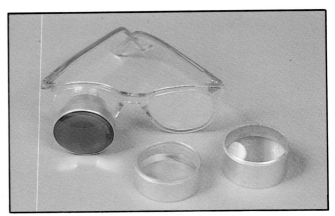

Figure 18. *Low visual aid. Spectacle telescope with adjustable lenses for distance or near viewing.*

Figure 16. *Corneal lens. Hard plastic lens smaller than the cornea.*

Figure 17. *Soft lens. Soft lens with the edge resting on the sclera.*

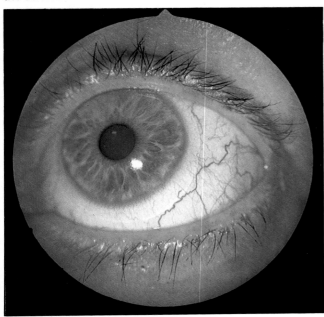

moving the lens which is washed and replaced. If a corneal abrasion is present the lens must be left out for at least 48 hours until the epithelium has healed. If the patient is wearing a soft lens do not use fluorescein dye until the lens has been removed, otherwise the lens will stain with the dye.

Infection is a rare hazard with hard lenses, but can occur with soft lenses. Minor defects in a soft lens can serve as a nidus for infection which may spread to involve the cornea.

Treatment is by removal of the lens, instillation of local antibiotic drops and referral to a contact lens specialist.

Low Visual Aids

The most important factor in obtaining good vision is adequate illumination. This applies to both distance and near vision. The moveable Anglepoise-type of light placed behind and slightly to one side of the head is ideal for reading or sewing.

A low visual aid consists of a magnifying system, the simplest being a hand-held magnifying glass. This may incorporate a light source like the popular 'map-readers'. The disadvantages are the small field of view, a short working distance, and the fact that only one hand is left free to hold the book or paper.

Spectacles which use the principle of the Galilean telescope (opera glasses) can achieve greater magnification without the short working distance, but still have only a small field of view. They may be adjusted for distance or near vision by altering the lens on the front of the glasses (Figure 18). □

thelium. The condition usually responds without treatment apart from removal of the lenses.

Corneal discomfort is usually the result of a small foreign body under the lens. This may be treated by re-

Inflammatory Lesions

Blepharitis

Blepharitis (inflammation of the lids) may be squamous or ulcerative. Both types are chronic conditions, and the squamous variety is more common.

Squamous blepharitis is marked by dandruff-like scales impaled on the lashes with an underlying eczematous reaction (Figures 1 and 2). The lid margins appear red and irritate, and the conjunctiva may appear injected. The scalp and eyebrows can be affected by seborrhoeic dermatitis with typical dandruff.

Treatment of the lids is by removal of the scales with damp cotton wool and the application of antibiotic and non-steroid ointment to the lid margins—chloramphenicol with oxyphenbutazone (Tanderil chloramphenicol). Frequent shampooing of the scalp may also be necessary.

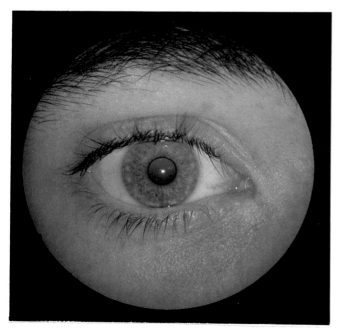

Figure 1. *Squamous blepharitis: redness of lid margins.*

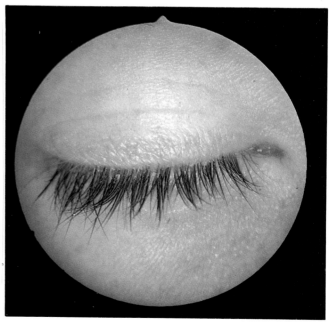

Figure 2. *Squamous blepharitis: white dandruff-scales at the base of the lashes.*

27

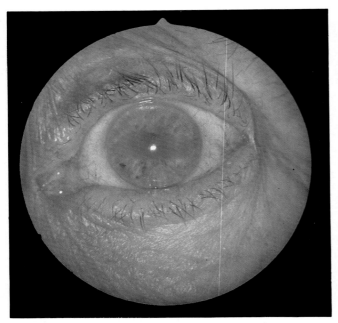

Figure 3. *Ulcerative blepharitis: multiple ulcers around the lashes.*

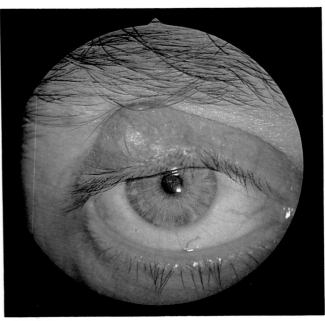

Figure 5. *Chalazion: swelling of the cyst is behind the lid margin.*

Figure 4. *Stye: small head of pointing abscess around the base of the lash.*

Figure 6. *Chalazion: internal granuloma developing from a ruptured meibomian gland.*

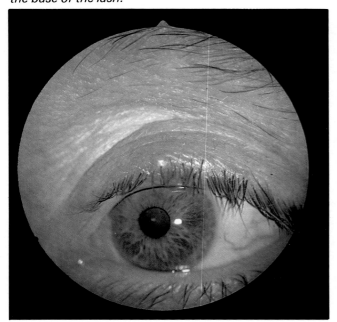

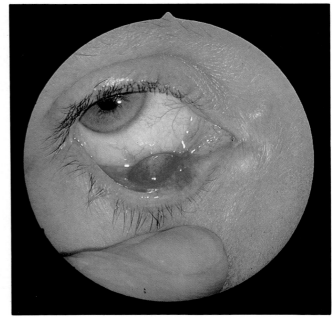

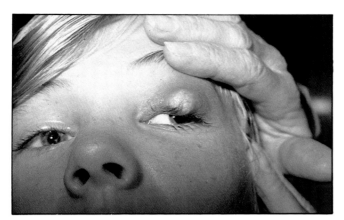

Figure 7. *Lid abscess.*

Figure 8. *Cellulitis: localized boil with surrounding redness and oedema of skin spreading to the upper and lower lids.*

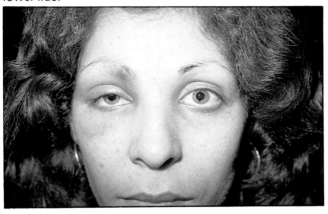

Ulcerative blepharitis is caused by a staphylococcal infection forming multiple abscesses of the lash follicles (Figure 3). The resulting ulcers, when healed, leave scarring of the lid margin with loss of the lashes or distortion (trichiasis).

Treatment with antibiotic ointment will prevent infection, but it may be necessary to remove any ingrowing lashes lest they abrade the cornea.

Stye

This is a localized abscess in a lash follicle caused by staphylococcal infection. It tends to point towards the lid margin along the line of the lash (Figure 4).

Treatment is seldom necessary as there is usually spontaneous discharge. Episodes of recurrent stye

formation should be treated with local antibiotic drops and the urine tested for sugar.

Chalazion

Retention of the secretion from a meibomian gland results in a localized swelling of the lid. This is usually directed away from the lid margin (Figure 5). Occasionally a granulomatous mass may be visible on the inside of the lid (Figure 6).

Treatment with local antibiotics and local heat is often successful in the early stages. If the swelling produces symptoms of pain or distortion of vision from pressure of the swollen lid, then incision and curettage is necessary.

Lid Abscess

This usually develops from an infected chalazion. It is very painful due to the localized swelling, and usually points towards the skin rather than the conjunctiva (Figure 7). Treatment is by surgical incision.

Cellulitis

Any infective lesion may cause cellulitis with pain, swelling, and redness of the surrounding skin. In the case shown in Figure 8 plucking the eyebrows has resulted in a local boil, which discharged spontaneously.

Orbital Cellulitis

Spread of infection from a nasal sinus can cause orbital cellulitis (Figure 9). The venous drainage from the face to the cavernous sinus makes the area around the eyes, nose and upper lip a danger zone because of possible retrograde spread of infection. This can result in cavernous sinus thrombosis. Treatment is by intensive systemic antibiotics.

Herpes Zoster Ophthalmicus

This is a viral infection involving the ophthalmic division of the trigeminal (fifth) cranial nerve, usually occurring in adults or the elderly.

The typical rash (Figure 10) is preceded by several days' pain over the eyebrow and there is generalized malaise and pyrexia. The skin eruption is over the frontal region, but rarely crosses the midline. The vesicles may turn to pustules due to secondary bacterial infection. Scabs form over the ruptured vesicles and when separated leave deep pitted scars.

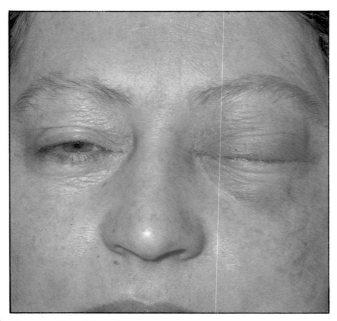

Figure 9. *Orbital cellulitis: patient unable to open painful swollen lids following spread of infection from a nasal sinus.*

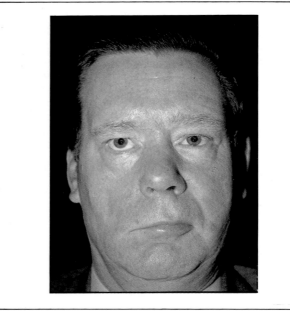

Figure 11. *Otic herpes zoster: right sided facial weakness with drooping of right lower lid.*

Figure 10. *Herpes zoster ophthalmicus: late stage with blisters crusting over. Lesions on the tip of the nose with ocular involvement.*

Figure 12. *Otic herpes zoster: attempted closure of the eyelids as in sleep leaving an area of exposed sclera and cornea.*

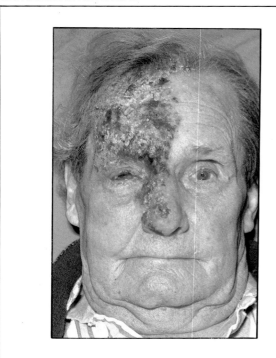

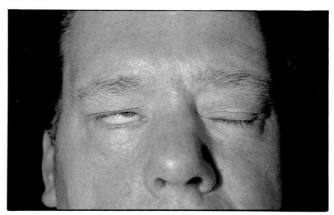

The neuralgic pain is very variable. It may be transient and diminish with the subsidence of the rash. However, it can be severe, radiating to the top of the head, and may last for years.

Eye involvement is frequent if there are vesicles on the side of the tip of the nose. About half of the cases of ophthalmic zoster develop ocular complications. Conjunctivitis, keratitis and iritis with glaucoma are relatively common, but gross swelling of the lids may prevent an adequate examination. If there is any doubt about the eye in such a case, referral to an ophthalmologist is essential.

If the ganglion of the facial nerve is involved, a Bell's palsy may be associated with vesicles in the external auditory meatus. Weakness of the facial musculature results in poor closure of the eye and exposure keratitis (Figure 11). The lower half of the cornea is exposed during sleep and the epithelium erodes (Figure 12). Treatment with antibiotic ointment may be sufficient but a lateral tarsorraphy to narrow the interpalpebral fissure may also be necessary (Figure 13).

Treatment for the ophthalmic lesion depends on the severity. Topical idoxuridine in dimethyl sulphoxide solution (Herpid) can be applied to the skin to prevent vesicle formation. Unfortunately, the diagnosis is rarely made until the skin changes are seen, by which time treatment is ineffective. Systemic antibiotics may be indicated to control secondary infection. Local steroids and systemic glaucoma therapy are needed for keratitis and iritis with raised intraocular pressure. Analgesics may be required when the neuralgia is severe.

Allergy

An allergy presents with extreme irritation around and in the eye with redness and swelling of the lids. There is an eczematous reaction with weeping and scaling of the skin (Figure 14). The conjunctiva may become swollen (chemosis) and inflamed. Conjunctival signs may be the only indication of an allergic reaction (Figure 15).

The commonest cause is a drug allergy, although cosmetics, rubber (elastic and gloves), metals (nickel clothes fasteners) and dyes (hairdressing and clothes) can cause contact dermatitis. Topical neomycin and atropine are the commonest causes. Rarely an allergy may be present to the preservatives in drops (phenyl mercuric nitrate or methyl hydroxy benzoate) or to the base in an ointment.

Treatment consists of the immediate discontinuance of the suspected drug, the application of antibiotic drops to the eye, and a steroid preparation to the skin.

Tumours

Xanthelasma

Xanthelasma is a yellowish-white plaque on the medial aspect of the upper or lower lids (Figure 16). It is caused by the deposition of lipids and is not therefore a true tumour. There may be an associated hyperlipoproteinaemia. The lesions may be single or may occur on all four lids. Treatment for cosmetic reasons is by surgical excision.

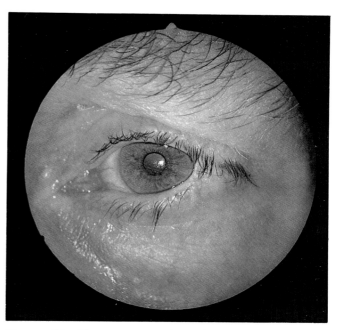

Figure 13. *Herpes zoster: lateral tarsorraphy may be necessary to narrow the interpalpebral fissure, to lessen exposure of cornea from facial weakness or to aid healing of corneal ulcers when affected by neuroparalytic keratitis.*

Figure 14. *Allergy: swollen shiny lids with serous discharge from allergy to atropine given for corneal ulceration.*

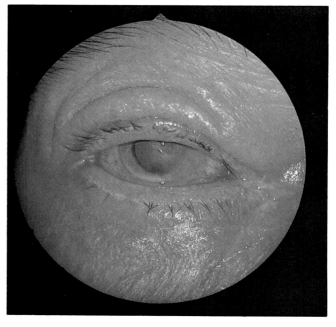

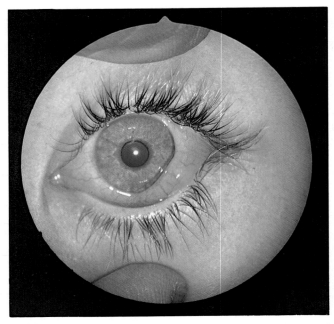

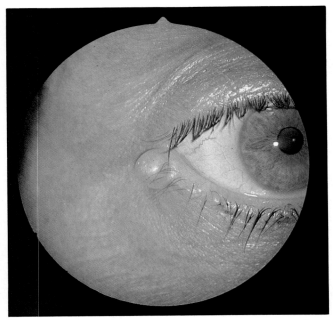

Figure 15. *Chemosis: gelatinous-like swelling of conjunctiva bulging over lower lid.*

Figure 17. *Marginal cyst: clear cyst arising in sweat gland.*

Figure 18. *Marginal cyst: sebaceous cyst.*

Figure 16. *Xanthelasmata: lipid deposits in the lids.*

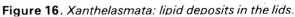

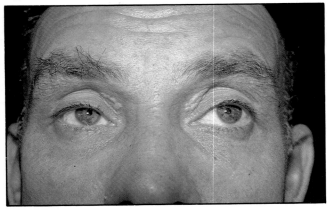

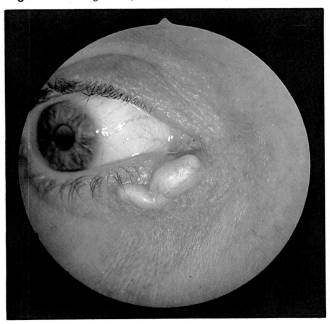

Cysts

Marginal cysts arise either from the glands of Moll (sweat glands), or the glands of Zeis (sebaceous glands). These lie in the lid margin associated with the lashes.

Sweat gland cysts are sometimes called clear cysts because they contain clear fluid (Figure 17). They can easily be pierced and opened with the cutting edge of a No. 1 needle.

Sebaceous cysts are whitish-yellow due to fat and cholesterol crystals (Figure 18). They can be 'shelled' out when small using a No. 1 needle, but may need more extensive excision when large.

Naevus

A naevus of the skin of the lids is usually of the raised type (Figure 19). The histology shows that it is benign and does not undergo malignant change. Treatment by surgical excision may be needed for cosmetic reasons.

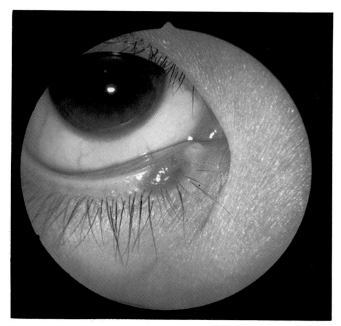

Figure 19. *Naevus: benign and slightly raised.*

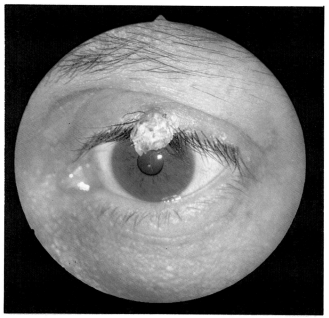

Figure 20. *Papilloma: horny excrescence.*

Papillomata

Simple papillomata are common around the eye. As they can reach quite a large size, early excision with cautery to the base is advisable (Figure 20).

Carcinomas

Basal cell carcinoma (rodent ulcer) is the commonest malignant tumour of the skin and occurs in the middle-aged or elderly. It is rare in dark skinned races, but is seen in Caucasians exposed to ultraviolet light in sunny climates. It presents two different types of lesion around the eye. The ulcerative form, which is the commonest, presents with a spreading invasive lesion (Figure 21). The central ulcer periodically scabs over and then breaks down and bleeds. In the cystic form, the lesion has a well defined pearl-coloured margin without any central ulceration (Figure 22). Both types tend to spread locally, but only slowly. They do not produce either local or distant metastases.

Treatment is by surgical excision, radiation or cryotherapy. All forms of treatment should be preceded by a biopsy to confirm the diagnosis. Surgical excision produces the best cure rate—95 per cent—but often at the expense of extensive plastic reconstruction of the lid. Inadequate excision can result in recurrence of the tumour (Figure 23). Radiation produces a high cure

Figure 21. *Basal cell carcinoma: typical spreading ulcerating lesion with raised edges, involving margin of lid.*

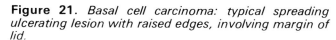

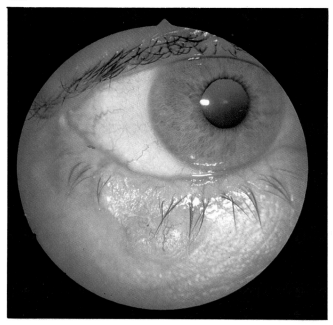

rate, but has added complications from local scarring, which can cause a watering eye due to loss of patency of the lacrimal drainage system. In the younger patient telangiectasia may occur (Figure 24). Cryotherapy using liquid nitrogen has produced some remarkable regression of tumours. However, it is still too early to assess this form of treatment.

Squamous cell carcinoma, although less common than basal cell carcinoma, is much more malignant. Local lymph nodes may be involved by metastases. The tumour may appear ulcerated, or it may develop the appearance of a papilloma (Figure 25). Treatment after biopsy is the same as for basal cell carcinoma, although the prognosis is poorer.

Deformities of the Lids

Entropion

The lid margin is turned inwards towards the eye (Figure 26). This is occasionally seen in babies due to fullness of the cheek and lower lid. It corrects itself spontaneously as the face grows. In the elderly the condition is caused by spasm of the orbicularis muscle, which is normally responsible for closing the eyelids. The cornea and bulbar conjuctiva are traumatized by the lashes. Secondary infection may supervene and can cause a corneal abscess.

In trachoma scarring of the conjunctival surface of the lids results in cicatricial entropion.

Temporary relief can be achieved by a piece of strapping, which is applied to the lid and then stuck down to the cheek to evert the lid margin (Figure 27). For permanent cure surgery is necessary.

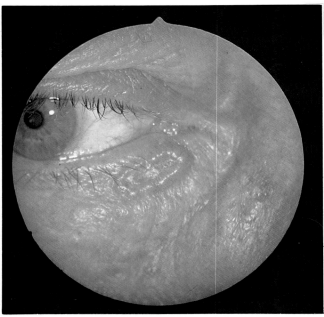

Figure 22. *Basal cell carcinoma: cystic type with no ulceration.*

Figure 23. *Basal cell carcinoma: recurrence of tumour at the junction of normal lid and the new lateral half of the lid from plastic reconstruction.*

Figure 24. *Basal cell carcinoma: complications of radiation treatment with telangiectasia of lower lid and loss of lashes.*

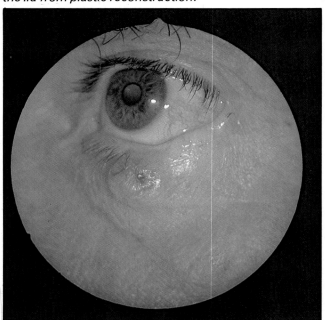

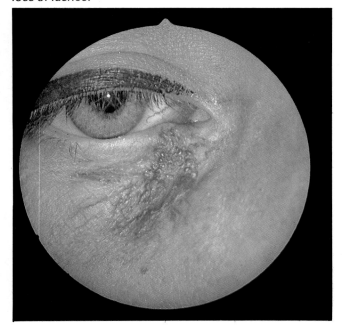

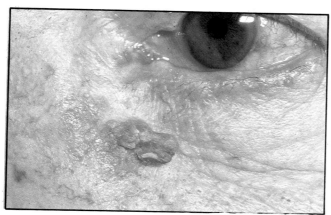

Figure 25. *Squamous cell carcinoma: papillomatous type with hyperkeratinization.*

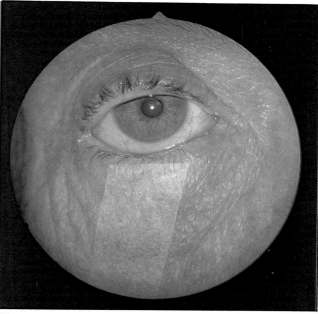

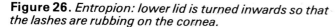

Figure 26. *Entropion: lower lid is turned inwards so that the lashes are rubbing on the cornea.*

Figure 27. *Entropion: emergency treatment with strapping to evert the lid.*

Figure 28. *Ectropion: medial two thirds of the lower lid are turned outwards. Thickening of inner surface tends to increase the deformity.*

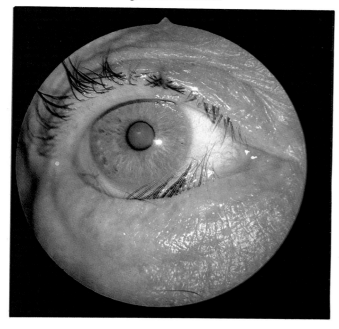

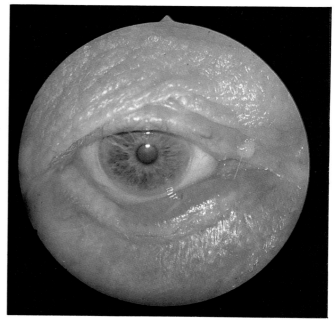

Ectropion

The lid margin is turned out from the eye (Figure 28). This is most commonly caused by atony of the orbicularis muscle. The drooping lower lid causes stagnation of tears with secondary infection and the exposed conjunctiva becomes thickened and inflamed.

Treatment with local antibiotics may control the infection in the early stages, but ultimately surgery is required.

Ectropion of the punctum of the lower lid is a common cause of watering eye (epiphora) in the elderly (Figure 29). Treatment is by cautery to the inside of the lid, to turn the punctum inwards.

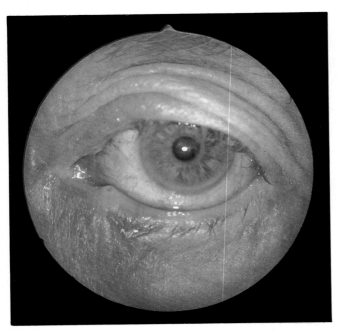

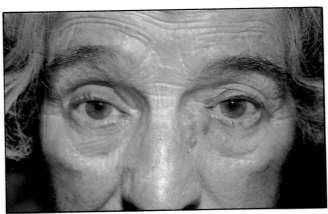

Figure 30. *Mucocele of lacrimal sac: a localized swelling is present below the right medial canthus. Normal tear drainage is absent.*

Figure 29. *Ectropion of punctum: the normal punctum opens on to the eyeball, here the punctum points upwards preventing the normal drainage of tears.*

Dacryocystitis

Watering of the eyes may be due to a blockage at the punctum, in the canaliculus or in the nasolacrimal duct.

Dacyryocystitis occurs when stagnant tears in the lacrimal sac become infected. When the condition is acute, there is a tender swelling with redness over the sac. In the chronic state a painless swelling of the sac occurs (mucocele) (Figure 30).

Treatment in the acute phase is with systemic antibiotics and drainage of pus from the sac by a simple incision. When a mucocele is present and the ducts cannot be opened by syringing, a dacryocystorhinostomy is necessary. This creates a new outflow from the sac into the nose by removing a portion of the bony lateral wall. In the elderly a dacryocystectomy to excise the sac is sometimes preferred as it is a simpler procedure.

The External Eye Part II

Conjunctival Cysts and Naevi

Conjunctival cysts

These appear as transparent swellings containing clear fluid and lie under the conjunctiva covering the sclera. They are either lymphatic or epithelial in origin.

Lymphatic cysts are small, sometimes multiple, dilatations of the lymphatic channels on the sclera. They rarely attain a very large size but may cause slight irritation.

Epithelial cysts may follow inflammation of the conjunctiva and are larger (Figure 1). Trauma to the conjunctiva or surgical incisions may lead to implantation of epithelial cells, which proliferate to produce a cyst (Figure 2).

Treatment is by excision if the swelling is large, but simple incision will often cure small cysts. This can easily be performed under local anaesthesia using a No. 1 needle.

Naevi

Small pigmented naevi of the conjunctiva are quite common. The amount of melanin they contain varies, some appearing black while others are almost colourless. They are benign.

Malignant change is indicated by a sudden increase in size, and enlargement of local blood vessels (Figure 3).

Pterygium

Pterygium appears as a triangular vascularized fleshy growth advancing from the conjunctiva on to the cornea (Figure 4). It occurs on the nasal side most frequently, but may be present on the temporal side. It gradually extends across the cornea, but does not cross the midline. The lesion may become inflamed and cause considerable discomfort. The condition is found more commonly in those who live in hot, dusty, sunny climates.

Treatment with local steroid drops will help inflammatory symptoms, but will not delay the extension of the lesion. Excision is indicated if the vision is

Figure 1. *Conjunctival cyst: large inflammatory bulla of conjunctiva.*

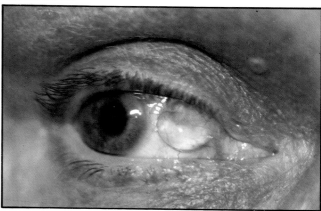

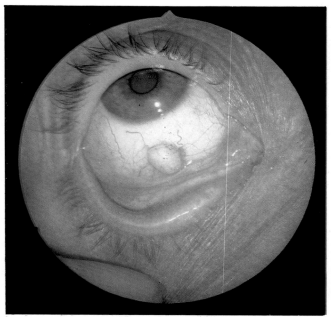

Figure 2. *Conjunctival cyst: discrete cyst following retinal detachment surgery.*

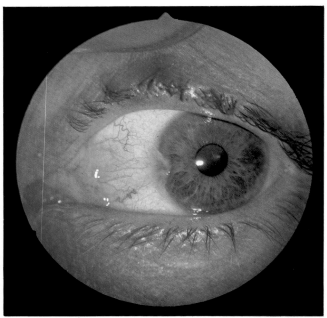

Figure 4. *Pterygium: a 'wing-like' growth extending across the cornea.*

Figure 3. *Conjunctival melanoma: increasing size indicates a change from a benign to a malignant condition.*

Figure 5. *Pinguecula: yellowish degenerative lesions on the exposed sclera adjacent to the limbus.*

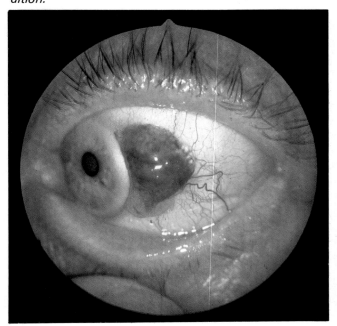

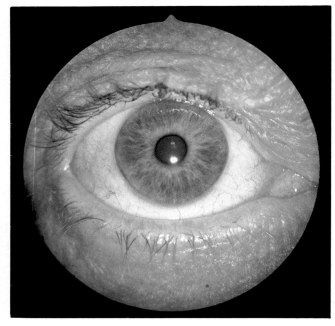

threatened, but it is usually advisable to operate when the lesion extends for more than a quarter of the corneal diameter. Several methods of surgical treatment have been described but the recurrence rate is high. Beta-radiation given after surgery may help to limit recurrences.

Pinguecula

Pinguecula is a triangular, yellowish area on the sclera adjacent to the cornea. Usually on the nasal side, it may also affect the temporal sclera (Figure 5). It is a degenerative condition and is an ageing process related to exposure.

Treatment is rarely necessary unless inflammatory changes occur, when astringent drops may help.

Conjunctivitis

Conjunctivitis is a common bilateral condition and is usually not serious. However, as some types like trachoma are potentially disastrous, it is wise to be cautious. Involvement, of only one eye must immediately arouse suspicion of the very dangerous conditions of acute glaucoma, acute keratitits and acute iritis. The diagnosis of conjunctivitis is made by the following symptoms and signs:

Figure 6. *Conjunctivitis: injection of superficial conjunctival vessels.*

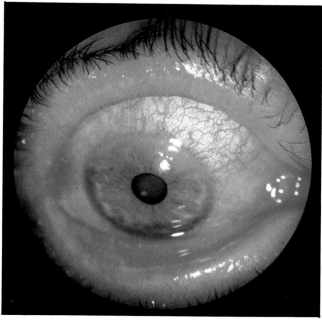

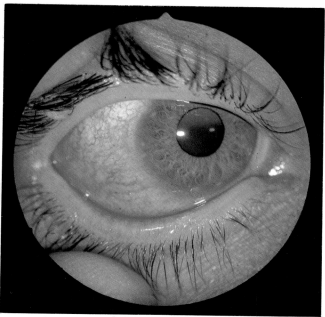

Figure 7. *Conjunctivitis: corneal involvment by white dots (infiltrates).*

1. Redness—injection of the superficial conjunctival vessels may be present over all or part of the eye and usually involves the lining of the lids. Individual vessels can be defined, in contrast to the diffuse redness seen in iritis (Figure 6).

2. Discharge—this may be purulent, mucopurulent or serous depending on the type and severity of the infection.

3. Discomfort and photophobia—a feeling of grittiness with increased watering may accompany dislike of bright light (photophobia).

Vision is not impaired except if the tear film is affected by the discharge.

Bacterial Conjunctivitis

This is the commonest variety of conjunctivitis, usually due to staphylococcal infection. The swollen lids, which stick together on waking, are lined by velvety thickened conjunctiva resulting from the formation of papillae. Corneal involvement can occur, with small infiltrates appearing near the limbus (Figure 7). These may enlarge or coalesce to form a greyish coloured ulcer (Figure 8). The cause is probably toxins produced by staphylococci.

Treatment consists of intensive local antibiotic drops by day and ointment at night. It is rarely necessary to confirm the diagnosis by bacteriological culture.

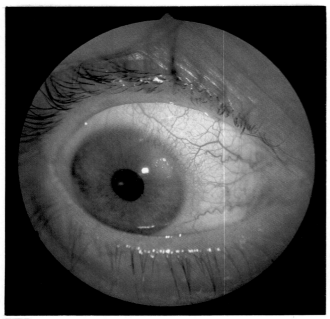

Figure 8. *Conjunctivitis: marginal keratitis with a greyish corneal ulcer adjacent to the limbus.*

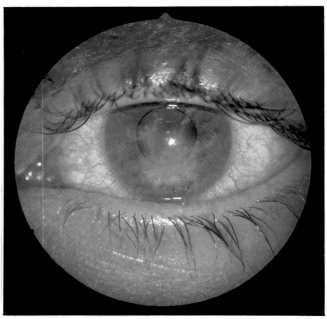

Figure 10. *Dendritic ulcer: branching pattern of the ulcer which stains with fluorescein dye.*

Figure 9. *Herpes simplex: primary infection with vesicle formation on the upper lids.*

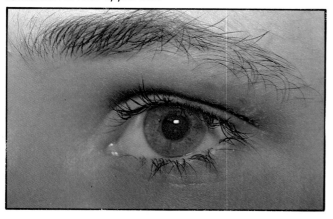

Gonococci

These cause ophthalmia neonatorum by direct infection from the mother at the time of birth. There is severe purulent conjunctivitis which can progress to corneal perforation and blindness. The condition is now rare in Europe and America, but is a common cause of blindness in the Indian subcontinent.

Treatment with local penicillin is the most effective.

Viral Conjunctivitis

This condition can be caused by several viruses, each giving a rise to a different clinical picture. Usually, the eyes are red and sore with a watery discharge. There is follicle formation in the conjunctiva due to aggregation of lymphocytes. Preauricular glands may become swollen and tender, and there may be pyrexia and pharyngitis.

Treatment is generally palliative but secondary infection requires antibiotics, and keratitis, if present, may be helped by steroids. Viral conjunctivitis is usually self-limiting but two types can cause particularly serious complications.

Trachoma

Trachoma caused by *Chlamydia trachomatis,* an organism intermediate between a virus and a Rickettsia, is the commonest cause of blindness in the world. A disease endemic in the Middle East, it has spread widely throughout the world and is common wherever poor social conditions and lack of hygiene prevail.

The clinical presentation varies, but at first there is usually a follicular conjunctivitis affecting mainly the upper lid. The cornea becomes involved by a pannus—a meshwork of blood vessels growing into the cornea.

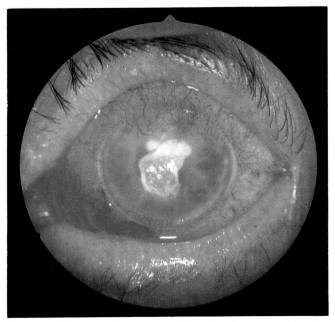

Figure 11. *Disciform keratitis: involvement of the deeper layers of the cornea by herpes simplex without epithelial ulceration.*

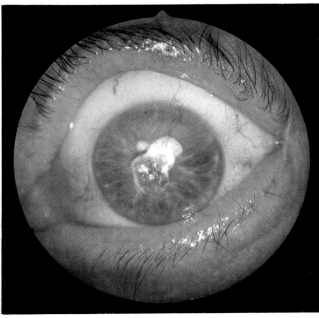

Figure 12. *Cholesterol degeneration: same case as Figure 11 after treatment. Central corneal scar contains a lipid deposit.*

from the limbus. A diffuse haziness of the cornea is present, due to infiltration by lymphocytes. After many months scarring of the inner surface of the lids results in distortion, with entropion of the lids. The constant trauma by the lashes on the diseased cornea, together with secondary bacterial infection, results in ulceration and gross corneal scarring.

Treatment using tetracycline ointment to the eyes and sulphonamides systemically can clear early cases. However, when the disease is advanced it may prove very resistant to treatment and surgical correction to the deformed lids may be necessary.

Herpes Simplex

The lesions of the herpes simplex virus can first appear as blisters on the lips (cold sores), around the eyelids (Figure 9) or on the cornea (dendritic ulcer). The primary infection occurs either in early childhood as a result of the affectionate kisses of an infected adult, or in the teens from the amorous advances of an affected lover.

The virus can remain latent for long periods, but may become active when the patient is debilitated or exposed to wind or sunlight. Recurrent episodes of virus activity most commonly produce the dendritic ulcer on the cornea (Figure 10). This has a branching pattern and

Figure 13. *Herpetic keratitis: scarring and vascularization of the cornea remaining despite treatment. Can only be removed by corneal grafting.*

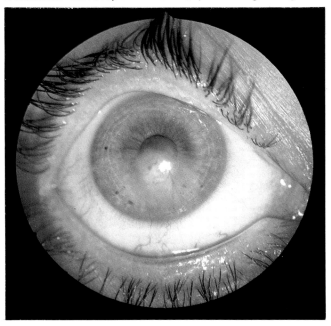

stains with fluorescein. Untreated, the lesion enlarges and may cover a large portion of the cornea.

Spread to the deeper layers of the cornea results in a disciform keratitis, producing more pain and blurring of vision (Figure 11). Subsequent attacks may only involve these deeper layers without producing an epithelial ulcer. Each attack leaves more scarring of the cornea, which may contain cholesterol crystals (Figures 12 and 13). Inflammation within the eye (uveitis) is common, and may be associated with a rise in intraocular pressure.

Treatment, using antiviral agents, should be carried out only by an ophthalmic department. The drugs in current use are idoxuridine (IDU), adenine arabinoside (Ara-A) and trifluorothymidine (F_3T). Mydriatic drops are used to overcome the pain of pupillary spasm and to prevent adhesions forming between the iris and the lens (posterior synechiae) when a uveitis is present. Steroid treatment should never be given except under the supervision of an ophthalmic department.

Corneal grafting may be indicated if there is poor vision as a result of scarring. Unfortunately, further recurrences of ulceration may attack the donor cornea.

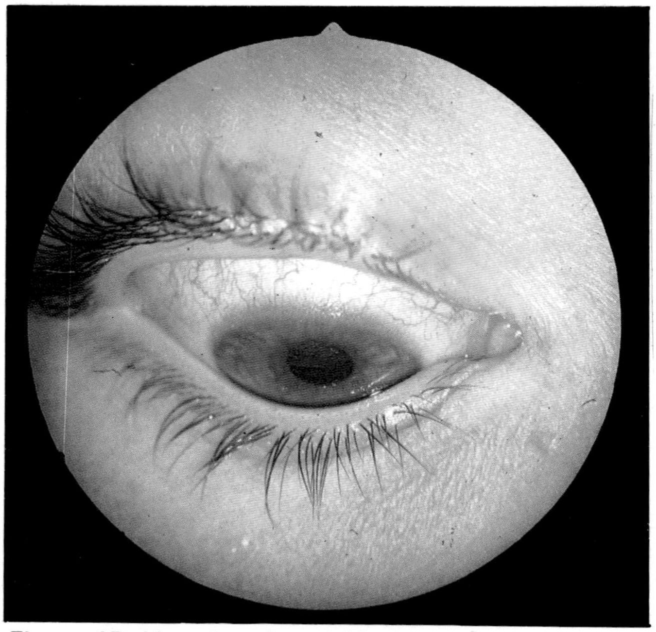

Figure 15. *Vernal conjunctivitis: involvement of cornea and limbus.*

Allergic Conjunctivitis

In addition to exogenous factors (drugs and cosmetics) already mentioned (see page 31), allergens can produce

Figure 14. *Vernal conjunctivitis: 'cobblestone' appearance from papillary overgrowth.*

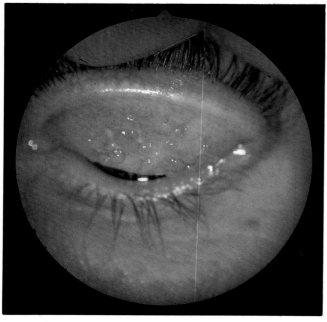

conjunctivitis. Hayfever is associated with intense irritation, with redness and swelling of the conjunctiva. Animals, mainly cats and horses, can produce a similar picture. Feather pillows and house dust have also been implicated.

Treatment is by avoidance of the allergen and local therapy with vasoconstrictors (Zincfrin, Antistin-Privine). Steroid preparations may be necessary in extreme cases. Desensitization may be indicated when the causative factors cannot be avoided.

Vernal Conjunctivitis

This allergic condition, also known as spring catarrh, affects the young and is rarely seen after the age of 40 years. It is seasonal in character and in the Northern hemisphere starts in May and June.

The upper lids are thickened by the formation of large papillae in the tarsal conjunctiva (Figure 14). The eyes irritate and there may be a slight drooping of the upper lids (ptosis). The discharge is slight but contains a high number of eosinophils, which are diagnostic of the condition.

When the limbus is involved gelatinous lumps appear in the upper half with localized redness of the conjunctiva (Figure 15).

Treatment with local antibiotics will control any

secondary bacterial infection. Steroid preparations produce considerable relief from symptoms and resolution of the ocular signs. However, the long-term use of these drugs should be avoided because of the risk of causing an increase in the intraocular pressure (steroid-induced glaucoma). Sodium cromoglycate two per cent drops (Opticrom) is a recently introduced preparation that produces considerable amelioration of the symptoms and signs of vernal conjunctivitis. Its use lessens the need for steroid treatment and in some cases it is possible to stop the use of steroids altogether.

Corneal Degenerations and Dystrophies

Arcus Senilis

Arcus senilis is an annular infiltration of lipid in the peripheral cornea. It is first seen as an arc at the inferior limbus, followed by another at the superior limbus, the two arcs extending to meet and form a complete ring. The 1 mm band is separated from the limbus by a clear zone of cornea (Figure 16).

The condition is an ageing process, but may be associated with a generalized hypercholesterolaemia. Occasionally, it is found in the younger age group and is then called arcus juvenilis.

Treatment is not required as the condition causes no visual abnormality.

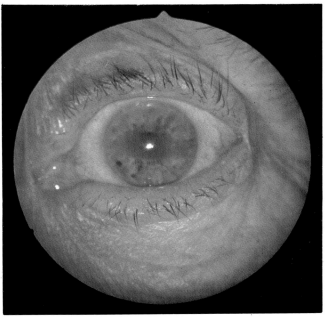

Figure 17. *Band degeneration: horizontal band of discoloured cornea occurring with chronic uveitis and Still's disease.*

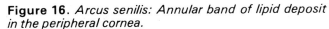

Figure 16. *Arcus senilis: Annular band of lipid deposit in the peripheral cornea.*

Figure 18. *Corneal dystrophy: mottled white appearance of cornea clearly seen against the black pupil.*

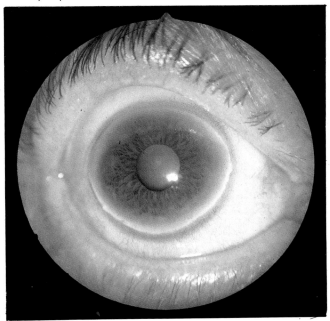

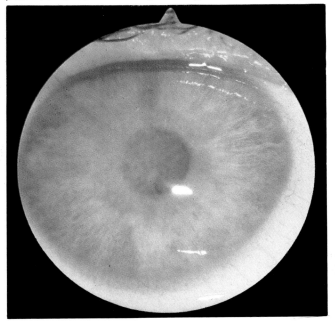

Band Degeneration

This condition is marked by the slow development of a greyish band, which extends from the limbus, on either side of the cornea. The two areas eventually meet so that the band extends across the full width of the exposed cornea (Figure 17). Occasionally the affected cornea may become white with the deposition of calcium salts. The condition may develop without any obvious precipitating factor, or it can occur as a result of a long-standing uveitis in adults or in Still's disease in children (polyarthritis with uveitis).

Treatment may be unnecessary if the vision is unaffected. The application of disodium ethylene diamine tetra-acetate (chelating agent) may clear the calcium deposits, but corneal grafting may be necessary.

Corneal Dystrophies

There are many hereditary degenerations of the cornea of unknown aetiology, which are grouped under the heading corneal dystrophies. Most of these affect the clarity of the cornea, and their classification is based on the anatomical distribution of the lesion in relation to the different layers of the cornea, and to the pattern of the degeneration (Figure 18). They are all relatively uncommon. Change in the shape of the cornea occurs with keratoconus (conical cornea). In this condition the cornea becomes thinned, and bulges forward in a cone-shape. This results in marked astigmatism which can best be corrected by contact lenses.

Treatment for all corneal dystrophies is by corneal grafting if the condition affects the vision. Superficial lesions can be treated by a lamellar graft in which only the outer layers of the cornea are replaced. Deeper lesions require a full-thickness or penetrating graft to remove the affected corneal tissues.   ☐

The Internal Eye

The portion of the inner eye that can be examined by the naked eye or using a magnifying glass is affected by several common conditions. Of these, glaucoma and cataract are so important that they warrant separate coverage and will be considered in future articles. This article deals with the inflammatory and infective diseases, together with tumours.

Uveitis

The uveal tract consists of iris, ciliary body and choroid, each of which can become inflamed separately or as part of a more generalized inflammation.

Iritis is the term for inflammation affecting the anterior portion of the uveal tract. It is also termed anterior uveitis or iridocyclitis. Choroiditis or posterior uveitis are terms for the inflammation of the choroid.

Uveitis is part of a systemic disorder or infection which may involve many other tissues. There is now known to be a strong association between particular human leucocyte antigens (HLA) and uveitis. Certain conditions having HLA 27 are associated with uveitis—for example ankylosing spondylitis, psoriasis, ulcerative colitis and Reiter's disease. Sarcoidosis accounts for less than 10 per cent of cases of uveitis. Uveitis can be caused by a wide range of infections—bacterial (tuberculosis and leprosy), viral (herpes simplex and herpes zoster), protozoan (toxoplasmosis) and treponemal (syphilis).

Infections producing choroiditis will be described in the section on the fundus.

Iritis

The clinical picture of iritis is of a rapid onset of pain, photophobia and blurring of vision. The eye is red, with the earliest changes appearing immediately adjacent to the limbus (ciliary injection, Figure 1). The anterior chamber contains numerous white cells which aggregate

Figure 1. *Uveitis: there is a pink blush appearing on the sclera around the limbus. The white areas on the cornea are caused by keratic precipitates. Posterior synechiae seal the pupil margin to the lens.*

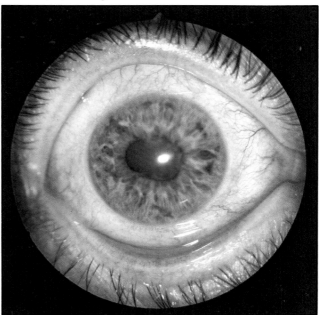

to form white dots (keratic precipitates, KP) on the corneal endothelium. Excessive production of inflammatory cells results in a hypopyon, when the cells form a sediment in the anterior chamber (Figure 2).

Leakage of protein from the dilated iris vessels can cause adherence of the iris to the cornea (anterior synechiae) or to the lens (posterior synechiae) (Figure 3).

The pupil is constricted, causing much pain from the spasm. Secondary glaucoma is a common complication caused by the blockage of the eye's drainage channels by protein and cells.

Investigations

Blood tests for syphilis, radiographs of the chest for sarcoidosis and of the sacroiliac joints for ankylosing spondylitis should be performed. However, nearly half of the cases of uveitis are found to have no obvious cause, despite widespread investigations.

Treatment

Treatment for an infective aetiology of iritis must be aimed at the cause. Antiviral agents for herpes simplex, penicillin for syphilis and antituberculous therapy for the rare cases of tuberculosis are necessary.

Anti-inflammatory treatment for the eye is given by local steroids, which can be in drops or ointment. The different forms of corticosteroid therapy will be discussed later in the series. Higher concentrations of steroids can be achieved by subconjunctival injection of the drug, or by systemic administration.

Mydriatic drugs are needed to relieve the pain from pupillary spasm and to prevent the formation of synechiae. In mild cases cyclopentolate one per cent (Mydrilate) or homatropine one to two per cent twice a day are sufficient, but atropine one per cent must be instilled three times each day in the more severe cases.

Antiglaucoma therapy for secondary glaucoma is by acetazolamide (Diamox) or dichlorphenamide (Daranide).

Prognosis

Iritis tends to be a chronic condition with relapses separated by weeks, months, or even, occasionally, years. The patient should be warned to seek the earliest possible treatment to minimize the complications.

Unfortunately the treatment is not without risk. Local steroids can cause a rise in intraocular pressure (steroid-induced glaucoma) and the long-term use of systemic steroids can result in the formation of posterior subcapsular cataract.

Hypopyon Ulcer

The healthy cornea forms a resistant barrier to penetration by infection into the inner eye. However

Figure 2. *Uveitis: generalized redness, keratic precipitates, hypopyon and posterior synechiae are all hallmarks of anterior uveitis.*

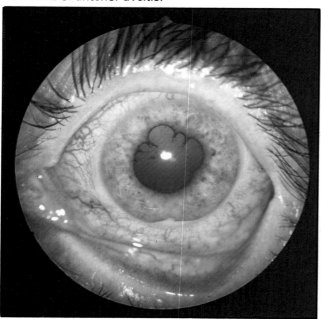

Figure 3. *Uveitis: posterior synechiae resulting from inadequate dilatation of the pupil.*

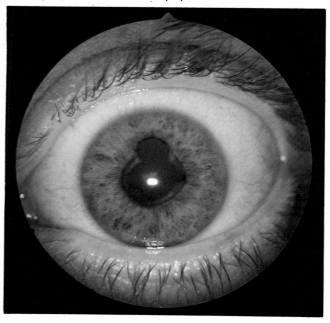

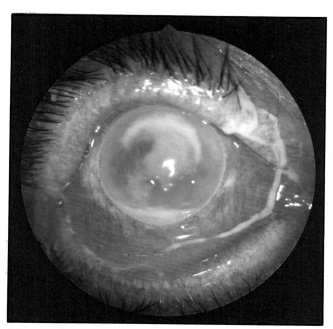

Figure 4. *Hypopyon ulcer: grossly infected eye showing corneal ulceration and abscess with hypopyon.*

severe corneal ulcers may result in changes within the eye.

Infection by pneumococci, gonococci or *Pseudomonas pyocyanea* can cause a hypopyon ulcer (Figure 4). The initial lesion may be minimal, but the infection spreads rapidly through the corneal stroma, and a corneal abscess may form (Figures 5, 6, 7 and 8).

Treatment with intensive local and systemic antibiotics can save the eye, but the vision is frequently severely affected due to scarring of the cornea and the formation of a cataract.

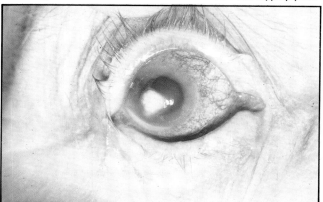

Figure 5. *Corneal abscess: localized area of corneal involvement with hypopyon in the anterior chamber.*

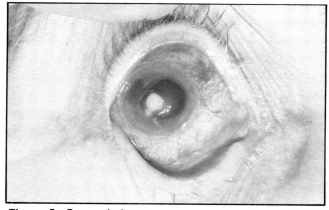

Figure 6. *Corneal abscess: same case as Figure 5 after 48 hours' treatment. Note absence of hypopyon.*

Figure 7. *Corneal abscess: localized area of abscess formation.*

Figure 8. *Corneal abscess showing the marked forward swelling of the cornea.*

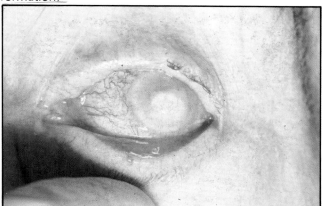

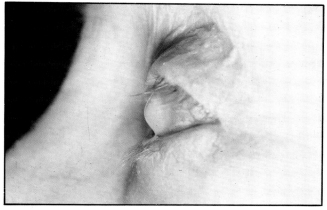

Tumours of the Anterior Uveal Tract

The only commonly seen tumours of the anterior uveal tract are the melanomata, which are either benign or malignant.

Tumours of the Iris

Benign Tumours

Collections of pigment known as iris freckles may be seen on the normal iris. Larger aggregations of pigment may develop at puberty. The lesions may be the size of a pin head or they may occupy a large segment of the iris. No treatment is required, except observation.

Malignant Tumours

Malignant tumours may develop from an existing benign lesion. A sudden increase in the size of the lesion, with distortion of the pupil and spread around the angle between the iris and the cornea, indicates probable malignancy (Figure 9).

Treatment is by local excision of the affected iris. However, as the tumour is very slow-growing a conservative approach can be taken in the older age group and simple observation substituted for radical surgery.

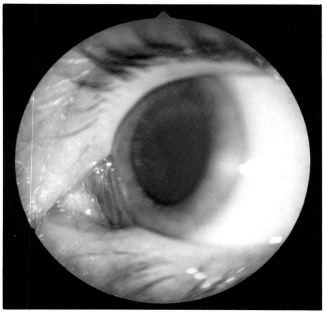

Figure 10. *Malignant melanoma of the ciliary body: raised pigmented lesion visible through the dilated pupil.*

Figure 9. *Melanoma of iris: small iris freckle with larger segmental area of malignant melanoma. There is pupillary distortion towards the melanoma. Gonioscopy showed very slow extension of the tumour around the angle of the anterior chamber.*

Figure 11. *Malignant melanoma of ciliary body, presenting with obvious extrascleral spread.*

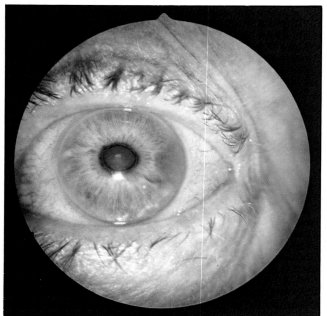

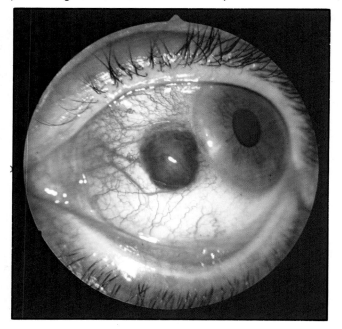

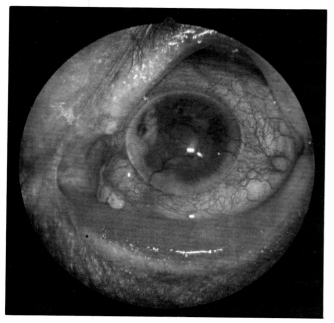

Figure 12. *Malignant melanoma of ciliary body: extension into the anterior chamber and early extrascleral spread. Treatment was refused by the patient.*

Tumours of the Ciliary Body

Benign lesions are rarely seen; they remain hidden behind the iris on account of their small size. However, malignant melanomata may be seen through the pupil on ophthalmoscopy (Figure 10) or may present by extraocular spread (Figures 11, 12 and 13).

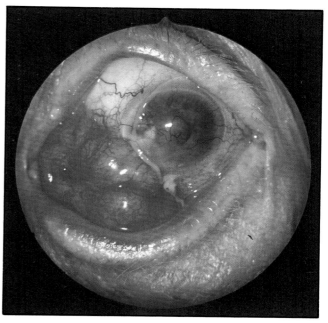

Figure 13. *Malignant melanoma of ciliary body: the same case as in Figure 12 seven months later, with further enlargement of scleral growth. The patient is still alive and well four years later.*

Treatment by excision is confined to the small tumours only. Enucleation of the eye is the only method when there has been extensive spread. Unfortunately, metastases can develop at an early stage in the disease and may remain quiescent for many years. Once the tumour has spread outside the sclera the mortality is considerably increased.

The Fundus Part I

It is possible to examine the fundus of the eye in detail because of the magnifying effect of the cornea and lens. A magnification of ×15 in the normal patient enables the optic disc, which is only 1.5 mm in diameter, to be seen in considerable detail.

In high degrees of myopia the magnification is greater, but the area of the retina that can be seen is smaller than normal; following cataract extraction the image size is much smaller but a larger area of retina is visible.

The Normal Fundus

In the normal fundus the colour of the retina depends on the amount of pigment in its pigmented epithelial layer and in the choroid. In the caucasian eye the retina is reddish-orange (Figure 1). This colour may have a superimposed pattern caused by areas of different pigment density. In the coloured races the denser pigment absorbs light and the fundus appears much darker (Figure 2). In myopia and albinism there is less pigment and the details of the choroidal vessels are visible (Figure 3).

The macular area, which lies temporal to the disc, is slightly darker than the surrounding retina. In the centre of the macula is the fovea, a small depression which is marked by a bright reflection of the ophthalmoscope light.

The Disc

The disc varies considerably in appearance although in any one person both discs are usually similar. Differences in the colour, shape, edge or vasculature may signify a pathological change or may just be part of the wide spectrum of normality. It is normally pink with a greyish-white depression—the physiological cup. This cup varies in shape, size and depth (Figure 4), and any

Figure 1. *Normal fundus in a caucasian.*

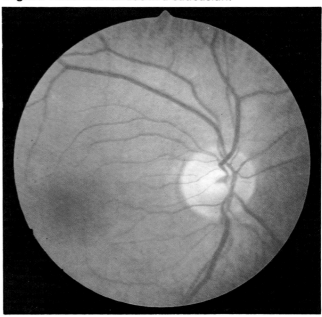

51

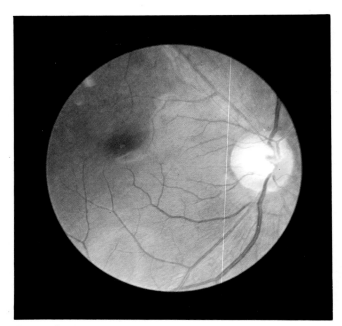

Figure 2. *Normal fundus in a coloured person.*

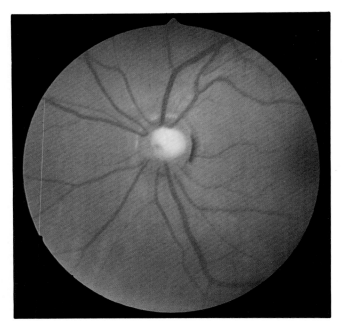

Figure 4. *Normal disc, showing broad physiological cup with a small pigmentary crescent.*

enlargement of the cup is one parameter used in the assessment of glaucoma. Disc pallor is associated with optic atrophy.

The disc is usually round or slightly oval vertically and not elevated above the surrounding retina. Apparent swelling of the disc may be seen in hypermetropia to give rise to pseudopapilloedema and is not pathological. Swelling may also be caused by local

inflammatory disease producing papillitis, or systemic conditions, such as raised intracranial pressure or malignant hypertension, which give rise to papilloedema.

The edge of the normal disc is well marked. Pigmentary crescents may be visible on the temporal side and may be accompanied by a crescent of white

Figure 3. *Normal fundus in myopia.*

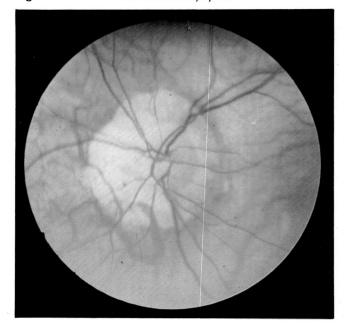

Figure 5. *Normal disc showing 'halo' found in myopia.*

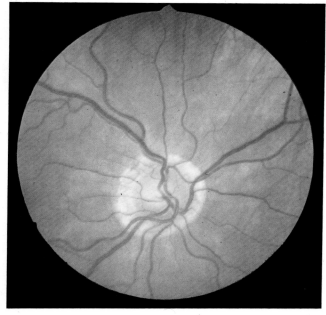

sclera in myopic eyes. Occasionally, this may extend around the whole circumference of the disc to form a white halo (Figure 5). Blurring of the edge of the disc usually accompanies papilloedema.

The retinal blood vessel pattern consists of arteries and veins which radiate from the disc to the four quadrants of the retina. There is as much variation in the arterial pattern as in the venous, but at the macular region all the vessels arch round, sending only small branches towards the avascular foveal area (Figure 6). Elsewhere, the arteries appear slightly narrower and a brighter red than the dark veins. At the disc the central retinal artery and vein lie in close association.

Arterial Obstruction

The retina, like the brain, is extremely susceptible to anoxia and even short periods of ischaemia can lead to irreversible changes.

Amaurosis Fugax

Amaurosis fugax presents as a sudden loss of vision in one eye, which may involve either the upper or lower field, and may be described as a shutter closing over the field of vision. Occasionally, the entire visual field may be lost. The visual loss lasts two or three minutes and there is then a slow improvement to complete recovery. The condition is painless.

Figure 6. *Fluorescein angiogram. Note the darker avascular area of the macula.*

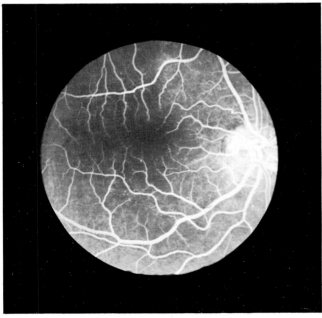

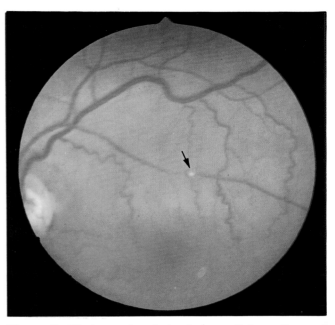

Figure 7. *Cholesterol embolus (arrowed) from diseased carotid vessels causing transient loss of vision.*

Amaurosis fugax is caused by emboli which originate in the heart as a result of valvular disease or mural thrombus, or from the internal carotid as a result of atheroma. These emboli impact in the retinal arteries but only partially interrupt the blood flow. Gradually, they disperse or pass to a more peripheral vessel and normal flow in the arteries returns. Retinal changes are rarely seen but an embolus may be found in a retinal artery (Figure 7).

The importance of the condition lies in its association with transient ischaemic attacks of the brain. Symptoms of weakness or anaesthesia of the opposite side of the body from the affected eye should be investigated with a view to vascular surgery (endarterectomy) to correct any carotid artery disease.

Retinal Artery Obstruction

Obstruction can occur either in the central retinal artery or in one of its branches. In either position the occlusion is complete so that an irreversible anoxia develops.

Central retinal artery obstruction causes a sudden complete loss of vision, and fundus changes develop within a few hours. The whole retina becomes whitish in colour, with the blood vessels barely visible because of their attenuation. The disc may appear swollen. There is a characteristic cherry-red spot at the macula where the choroid can be seen through the thin retina (Figure 8). Occasionally, the central vision may be spared if there is a separate artery to the macular area (Figure 9).

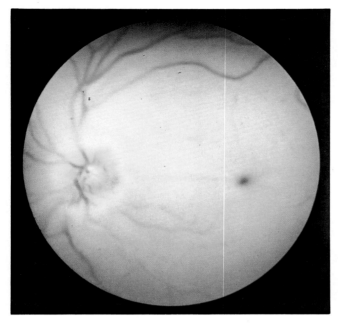

Figure 8. *Central retinal artery occlusion: total loss of vision with white oedematous retina, narrowed vessels and cherry-red macular spot.*

Branch retinal artery obstruction produces symptoms similar to amaurosis fugax but without the spontaneous recovery. The fundus changes involve only the part of the retina supplied by the occluded vessel, and the effects of the anoxia within this area are similar to those

Figure 9. *Central retinal artery occlusion: central vision is spared due to a separate blood supply to the macula but peripheral vision is lost.*

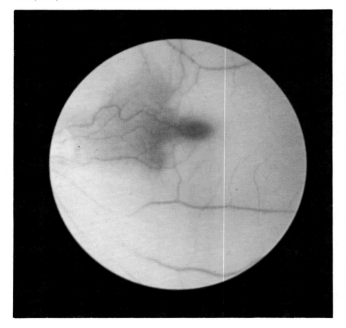

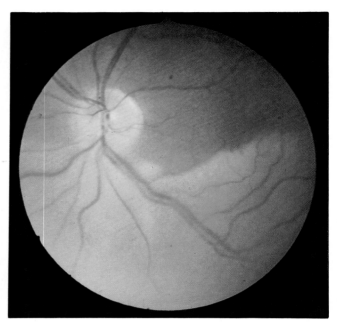

Figure 10. *Branch retinal artery occlusion: oedema is limited to the lower half of the retina, causing an upper half defect in the visual field.*

of a central artery occlusion (Figure 10).

Arterial occlusion may be caused by arteriosclerosis with hypertension, embolism from the heart or carotid system and temporal arteritis.

Treatment is usually unsuccessful as the ischaemia is

Figure 11. *Central retinal vein occlusion: flame-shaped haemorrhages cover the retina and mask the disc.*

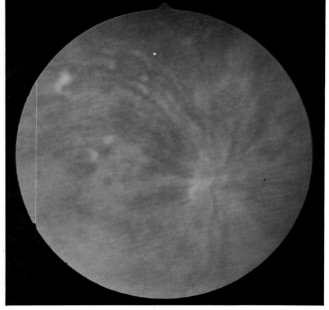

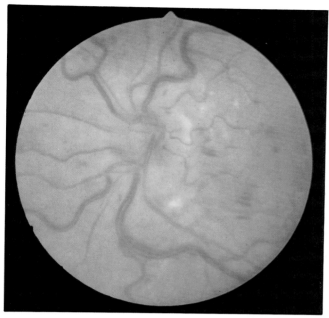

Figure 12. *Central retinal vein occlusion: partial obstruction has caused venous dilation but minimal haemorrhages. The visual prognosis is better than in complete occlusion.*

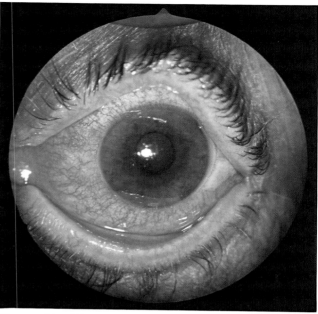

Figure 14. *Thrombotic glaucoma: dilated vessels on the iris (rubeosis iridis) are associated with raised intraocular pressure causing a painful red eye.*

severe by the time the diagnosis has been made. However, lowering the intraocular pressure with intravenous acetazolamide and massage of the globe may help to dislodge an embolus.

Figure 13. *Branch retinal vein occlusion: there are retinal haemorrhages distal to the site of venous obstruction.*

Venous Obstruction

Obstruction of a retinal vein produces a back pressure resulting in retinal haemorrhages. As in the arterial system, the occlusion may affect either the central retinal vein or one of its branches.

Figure 15. *Venous occlusion, showing late development of hard exudates and macular oedema.*

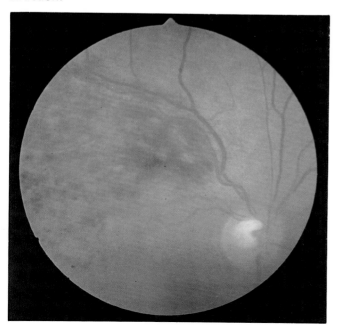

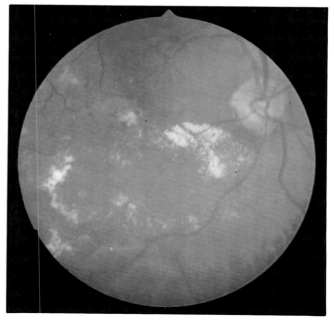

Central retinal vein obstruction presents less dramatic symptoms than those of arterial involvement. Although vision fails, its loss is neither so sudden nor complete. The fundus changes are usually severe. Haemorrhages are widespread throughout the retina. The deeper round-shaped haemorrhages àre masked by the superficial flame-shaped variety caused by leakage of blood in the nerve fibre layer of the retina. The retinal veins are grossly dilated and loop in snake-like fashion in and out of the oedematous retina (Figure 11). Scattered soft exudates may occur, and the disc is often swollen and partially obscured by haemorrhages. Less florid cases may have few haemorrhages but dilated tortuous veins (Figure 12).

Branch retinal vein obstruction may give rise to only slight visual symptoms if the peripheral retina alone is involved. When the macular area is affected, a marked drop in the visual acuity occurs. In the fundus, multiple haemorrhages are produced beyond the site of the venous obstruction, usually at an arteriovenous crossing (Figure 13). The superior temporal vessel is the most commonly affected.

The causes of venous obstruction are arteriosclerosis with hypertension, diabetes, chronic glaucoma and increased viscosity of the blood, such as occurs in polycythaemia.

The prognosis for central vein occlusion is variable. In some cases there is almost complete resolution with a good visual result, while in 20 per cent of cases the haemorrhages persist, leading to thrombotic glaucoma and loss of the remaining vision (Figure 14). Fluorescein angiography can indicate those patients who are likely to develop complications.

Branch vein occlusion can clear completely if an effective collateral circulation develops. However, neovascularization, macular oedema and exudates may form to threaten the vision (Figure 15).

Treatment with light coagulation has a beneficial role in some cases with new vessels and macular oedema where previously no effective treatment was available. □

The Fundus Part II

Macular Disease

The macular area is the most sensitive part of the retina for photopic or daylight vision, and is represented in the occipital lobes by the largest area on the visual cortex. Macular disease is one of the commonest causes of blindness and results in the loss of the central visual field.

Figure 1. *Senile macular degeneration: patchy pigmentary change occurs only at the macula.*

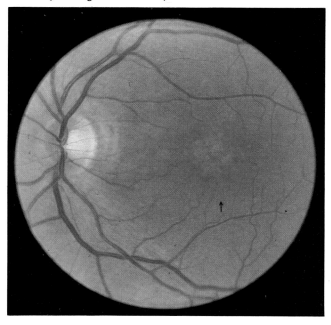

The symptoms vary, depending on the aetiology. A gradual deterioration in the visual acuity is the commonest symptom, but sudden loss may occur following a macular haemorrhage. Distortion of straight lines, micropsia (objects appearing smaller than normal) and alteration in colour vision may also be noticed.

Senile Macular Degeneration

This condition is a change that accompanies ageing and is the commonest reason for registration as blind in Great Britain. Visual acuity is gradually impaired in one and then both eyes, and the macula appears mottled with patchy pigmentation (Figure 1). There may be surrounding drusen which are seen as yellowish white spots (Figure 2). Drusen may occur without any macular degeneration and may be seen in the peripheral retina, sharply defined by a pigment outline. Occasionally, drusen are found in the optic disc (Figure 3).

Disciform Degeneration of the Macula

This condition occurs as part of the senile change that results from arteriosclerosis, and the central vision fails suddenly as a result of a choroidal haemorrhage. The macula appears greyish and elevated in the early stages, but after several months the area becomes scarred and turns white (Figure 4). The condition is usually bilateral, but there is an interval between the onset in the two eyes.

Fluorescein angiography shows the development of

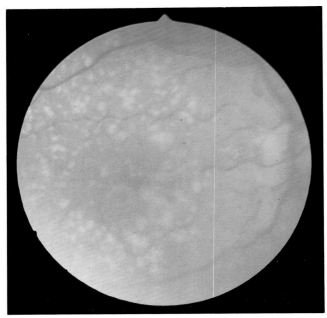

Figure 2. *Drusen, appearing here as scattered yellow spots, may occur without any disturbance to central vision.*

an area of neovascularization, which may be treated in the early stages by photocoagulation. However, no treatment is possible by the time an organized scar has formed.

Figure 3. *Drusen, seen here as white spots in the disc, may be associated with field defects similar to chronic glaucoma.*

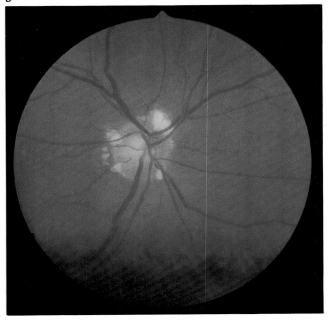

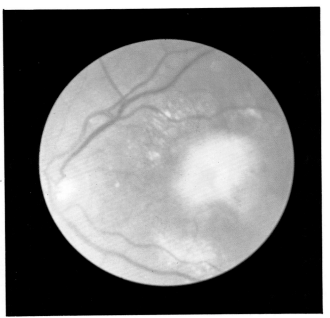

Figure 4. *Disciform degeneration of the macula, showing an organized white scar, formation of which renders the loss of central vision irreversible.*

If one eye is affected the patient should be advised to report any symptoms of visual distortion in the fellow eye. The results of early treatment are encouraging.

Macular Haemorrhage

Retinal haemorrhage is usually associated with vascular disease (arteriosclerosis, diabetes and hypertension) or trauma.

Haemorrhage at the macula can extend forward and become localized between the vitreous and the retina, to form a subhyaloid haemorrhage. This has a characteristic hemispherical shape with a straight upper edge (Figure 5). The condition occurs with trauma or when arterial disease exists. Complete resolution with full recovery of central vision can occur when the cause is traumatic, but a permanent central field defect may persist if the haemorrhage is longstanding.

Myopic Degeneration

The fundus may show marked degenerative changes in myopia. In addition to the crescent around the disc, there is generalized thinning of the choroid and retina so that white patches of bare sclera are visible at the posterior pole. A sudden permanent loss of central vision may occur with the development of a Foster-Fuch spot at the macula (Figure 6). This appears as a

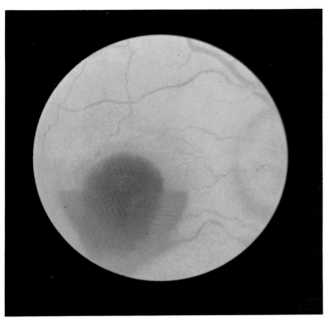

Figure 5. *Subhyaloid haemorrhage: blood from a macular haemorrhage has collected between the retina and the vitreous giving a straight upper border.*

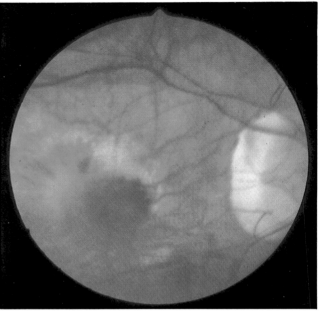

Figure 6. *Myopic degeneration: dark haemorrhagic spot at the macula causing sudden loss of central vision.*

dark circular area which results from a choroidal haemorrhage with changes in the pigment epithelium.

Retinitis Pigmentosa

This is a degenerative condition affecting the light-sensitive layer of the retina, particularly the rods. It presents in childhood and may progress to blindness in middle age. Early diagnosis can be obtained using the electroretinogram, but the condition is untreatable. The characteristic symptoms are defective vision at night and progressive limitation of the peripheral visual field (Figure 7).

Changes in the fundus are attenuation of the retinal vessels, pigmentary changes (bone-corpuscle shapes in the midperiphery) and a waxy pallor of the optic disc (Figure 8). The condition has a definite hereditary tendency with a dominant, recessive or sex-linked trait, but genetic counselling can only be given when the exact type of pedigree is known.

Choroiditis

Inflammation of the choroid may be part of a generalized uveitis in which the signs affect the whole of the eye (anterior and posterior uveitis), or it may present with changes found only in the fundus.

Anterior uveitis was discussed in the chapter on the internal eye (Chapter 6). Posterior uveitis is caused by the parasitic infestations toxoplasmosis, toxocariasis and occasionally histoplasmosis, and more rarely by sarcoidosis and syphilis.

Toxoplasmosis

This protozoal disease is usually acquired congenitally when the mother has a subclinical infection. Evidence of the disease may be present in the first six months of life, especially with a macular lesion which can cause a squint. Alternatively, the condition may only be discovered on routine eye examination many years later.

The fundus has scattered white areas with deeply pigmented sharp edges (Figure 9). They vary in size from about half the diameter of the optic disc to several times its width. These inactive lesions may occur anywhere in the fundus; when they are found adjacent to the disc the condition is called juxtapapillary choroiditis (Figure 10). In the active phase of toxoplasmosis the overlying vitreous is hazy and the visual acuity falls dramatically.

Diagnosis is helped by serological tests, but the condition is resistant to treatment. Systemic and local corticosteroids may suppress the inflammatory signs of toxoplasmosis.

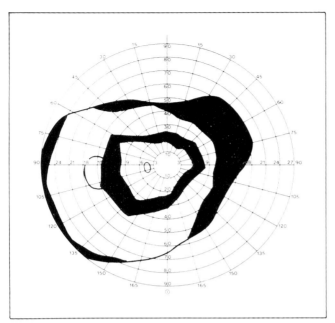

Figure 7. *Retinitis pigmentosa: characteristic loss of visual field in a 25-year-old man complaining of night blindness.*

Toxocariasis

This condition is caused by the larvae of an intestinal worm found in dogs. It most commonly affects children who have contact with puppies or dogs that have not regularly been dewormed.

The ocular signs appear either as a granuloma or as a

Figure 9. *Toxoplasmosis: a discrete white area with pigmented edge typical of the inactive phase of the condition.*

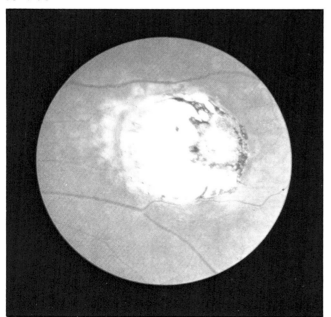

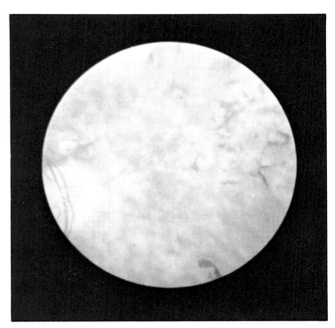

Figure 8. *Retinitis pigmentosa, showing attenuation of vessels, pigmentary changes and pallor of the disc.*

chronic endophthalmitis. The whitish granuloma is usually found in the macular region (Figure 11). It must be differentiated from a retinoblastoma; the latter tends to increase in size and on a radiograph may show calcification.

The chronic endophthalmitis may present with a generalized uveitis, with haziness of the vitreous. A

Figure 10. *Toxoplasmosis: inactive lesions occurring next to the disc.*

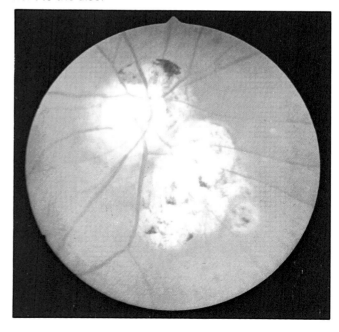

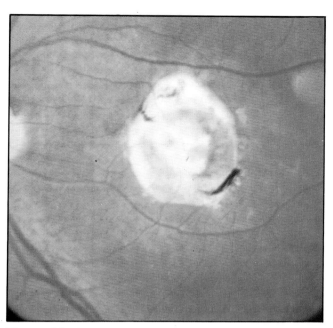

Figure 11. *Toxocariasis: a white granuloma mimicking a retinoblastoma.*

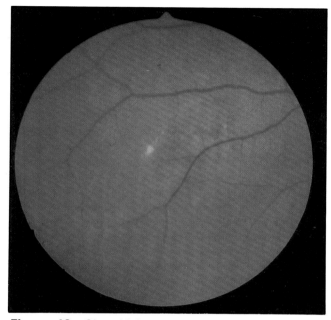

Figure 13. *Choroidal naevus: a typical benign, flat, greyish lesion with feathery edges.*

white mass may be visible in the extreme periphery of the fundus (Figure 12).

Treatment is difficult; no drug is effective against the larva, but corticosteroids can limit the inflammation.

Figure 12. *Toxocariasis: a painting of a fundus with a peripheral white ring of inflammation in a presumed case of toxocariasis. Scarring around the disc has caused a slight reduction of visual acuity.*

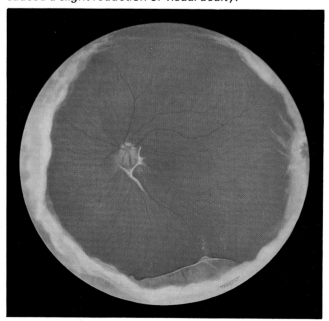

Choroidal Tumours

Benign Naevus

This is a bluish-grey flat lesion occurring at the posterior pole of the eye (Figure 13). It is about the same diameter as the disc, and the surface of the lesion may have white dots. The tumour is shown to be benign by its unchanging nature. It gives rise to no symptoms and does not require treatment.

Malignant Melanoma

This is the commonest of the malignant tumours of the uveal tract. It presents in the fifth decade either as a chance finding on routine ophthalmoscopy or as a result of visual field defects. The lesion is raised, with a variable amount of pigmentation. The tumour rapidly increases in size and may break through Bruch's membrane and raise the retina with a mushroom-like extension (Figure 14). There may be an associated exudative detachment of the retina; this may be quite separate from the tumour in the lower half of the fundus.

The tumour gradually fills the globe causing glaucoma and eventually extraocular extension. Metastases can develop even in the early stages of the condition.

Enucleation of the eye has been the standard method of treatment, but treatment of small lesions with light coagulation and radiation has had some success. In the elderly with good vision the tumour is best observed as

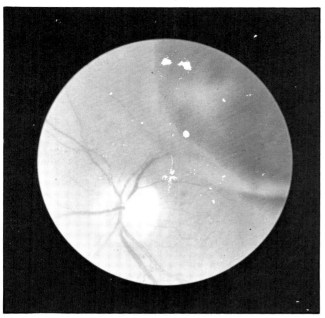

Figure 14. *Choroidal malignant melanoma: a heavily pigmented tumour enlarging into the eye and meta- stasizing most commonly to the liver.*

the growth may be very slow. Blood-borne metastases may not become evident for many years.

Retinal Detachment

In retinal detachment the light-sensitive rods and cones

become separated from the underlying pigment epi- thelium. The function of the photoreceptors depends on the pigment epithelium, so that early surgery to restore the normal anatomy is vital.

Detachment of the retina occurs when a retinal hole is formed by the traction of the vitreous on a weak area in the retina. This weakness is commonest in the upper temporal quadrant and is more frequent if the eye is myopic.

Symptoms and Signs

The symptoms of detachment are flashing lights, and floaters which may appear as dots or cobwebs. When the retina becomes detached the appearance of a curtain or shutter passing across the field of vision may be noticed. A small peripheral detachment may pass un- noticed, whereas detachment of the macula causes immediate loss of central vision.

The signs of retinal detachment are the loss of the normal red reflex. The affected retina is grey and the retinal vessels appear darker than normal (Figure 15). Tears in the peripheral retina may be visible.

Treatment

Treatment consists of bed rest followed by appropriate surgical techniques to appose the two layers of the retina. Silicone sponge is used to indent the sclera

Figure 15. *Retinal detachment: a raised grey area of retina extending from the periphery to the edge of the macula, with a single round tear.*

Figure 16. *Retinal detachment: the same case after surgery. The white areas formed by cryotherapy, used to seal the defect in the retina.*

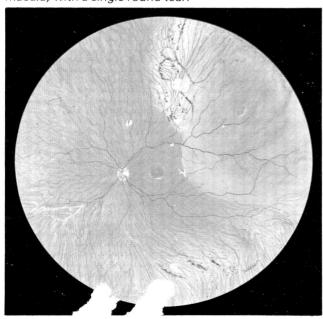

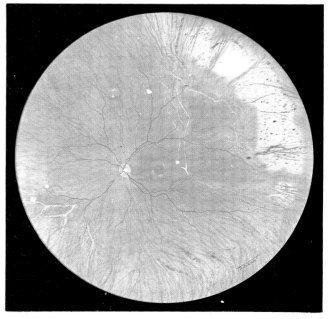

towards the retina and cryotherapy is applied to achieve adhesion between the layers (Figure 16).

Prophylactic treatment of weak areas of retina, using cryotherapy or light coagulation, can prevent the development of retinal tears and subsequent retinal detachment.
□

9

Trauma to the Eye Part I

The exposed position of the eye makes it very susceptible to injury. While the bony orbital margin provides some protection from blunt injury by large objects, the lids are not an effective barrier to small sharp objects.

Head Injuries

Relatively mild head injuries can give rise to cranial nerve damage, which may have ocular complications. The third, fourth and sixth cranial nerves may be affected, causing a paralytic squint. This produces double vision in the direction of gaze of the affected muscle. For example, a right sixth nerve lesion will cause diplopia on looking to the right. Minor degrees of horizontal muscle imbalance usually settle spontaneously, but vertically acting muscle weakness may cause lasting symptoms. This is particularly true of trauma to the fourth cranial nerve which supplies the superior oblique muscle.

Weakness of the facial muscles caused by seventh cranial nerve involvement may cause inability to close the eye (Figure 1) and subsequent exposure keratitis. This usually resolves spontaneously, but treatment is needed if corneal ulceration develops.

Facial Lacerations

Road traffic accidents account for many of the injuries to the globe and its adnexae. Facial lacerations caused by windscreen glass, when a seat belt is not worn, are usually horizontal. Sometimes, a double row of lacerations occurs high on the forehead. If the cuts are lower they may involve the lids and the eye balls (Figure 2). Profuse bleeding may mask serious damage to the globe and careful examination under general anaesthetic is advisable.

Figure 1. *Right-sided facial weakness following a road traffic accident.*

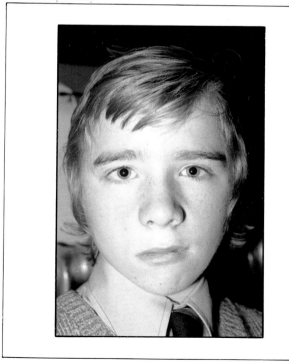

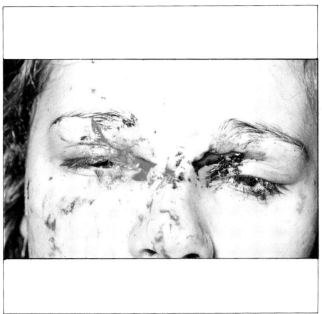

Figure 2. *Facial lacerations from a shattered wind-screen, involving full thickness of the upper lids.*

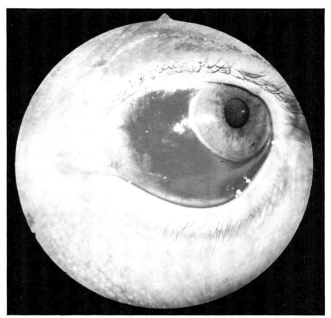

Figure 4. *Subconjunctival haemorrhage: haemorrhage originating from intraorbital damage covering the entire conjunctiva.*

Simple lacerations of the lids with no loss of tissue may be sutured under local anaesthesia. If the lid margin is involved accurate apposition must be achieved to avoid the formation of 'steps' or notching of the margin.

Figure 3. *Subconjunctival haemorrhage: localized area of bright red blood.*

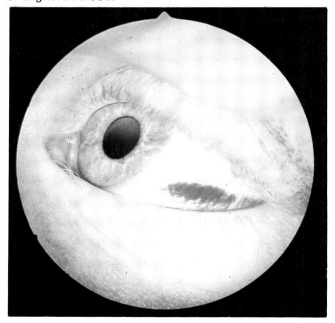

When the medial third of the lid is involved, the lacrimal ducts are at risk. If the upper canaliculus becomes occluded by subsequent scar tissue, the lower canaliculus can cope with the normal tear drainage. Blockage of the lower canaliculus, however, results in a permanent watering eye. Such blockage is prevented by the insertion of a fine polythene tube which acts as a splint, and prevents scarring and narrowing of the tear duct.

Subconjunctival Haemorrhage

This can occur spontaneously in the elderly, or it may be the result of ocular trauma. The subconjunctival blood retains a bright red appearance and does not undergo the colour changes seen in a subcutaneous bruise (Figure 3). Absorption of the blood occurs within two weeks and no treatment is required.

If the posterior border of the haemorrhage cannot be seen (Figure 4) then possible orbital damage should be suspected.

Orbital Fractures

A 'blow-out' fracture of the floor of the orbit occurs when the orbital contents are forced down into the maxillary antrum. This can occur with a blunt injury such as a blow from a fist. The inferior rectus and

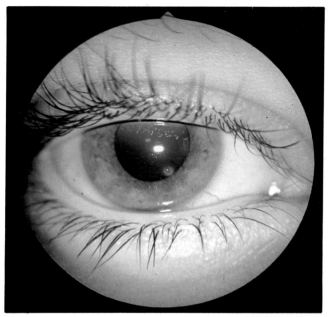

Figure 5. *Corneal foreign body.*

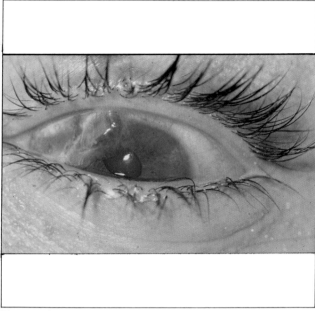

Figure 6. *Corneal laceration: full thickness laceration with iris prolapse. The pupil is oval shaped and drawn towards the wound.*

oblique muscles become trapped, so limiting elevation of the eye. Radiography shows an opaque antrum with a defect in the floor of the orbit. Full recovery of ocular movements usually occurs without recourse to surgery.

Corneal Injury

Corneal abrasions and superficial foreign bodies cause pain and watering of the eye. Large abrasions are usually obvious; the application of fluorescein allows smaller lesions to be seen more easily.

A foreign body on the cornea is usually readily visible (Figure 5), but one in a subtarsal position may be missed unless the lid is everted. It is possible to remove a superficial foreign body with a swab or sterile needle, after instillation of a local anaesthetic such as oxybuprocaine (Minims Benoxinate). Occasionally a rust ring remains which, if small, can be left.

Embedded foreign bodies should be dealt with by a specialist; attempted removal by an unskilled shaky hand may at best lead to corneal scarring and at the worst to corneal perforation.

A defect in the corneal epithelium is treated by instillation of antibiotic ointment, and padding. A short-acting mydriatic such as cyclopentolate (Mydrilate) may help to relieve any pain from pupillary spasm.

Chemical burns require urgent treatment with large volumes of water to dilute the agent. Acid burns cause less extensive injuries than alkaline burns, which tend to penetrate the eye causing marked iritis and cataract formation.

Full-thickness lacerations of the cornea or sclera pose a serious threat to the eye because intraocular contents can be lost and infection can readily enter (Figures 6 to

Figure 7. *Corneal laceration: same eye as in Figure 6 after surgery. The prolapsed iris has been excised to form a broad iridectomy.*

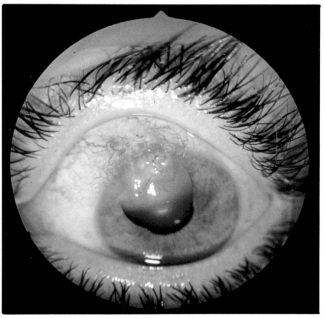

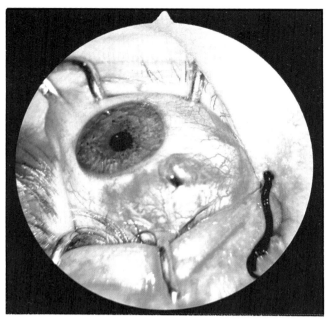

Figure 8. *Scleral laceration: full thickness star-shaped laceration with loss of vitreous and herniation of dark choroidal tissue.*

Figure 10. *Hyphaema: blood level in the lower half of the anterior chamber.*

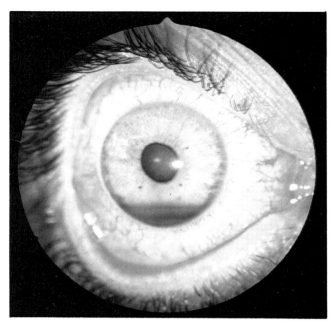

Hyphaema

9). The eye should be covered by a pad, without any local medication, and the patient transferred for specialist supervision.

Blunt injury to the eye may cause rupture of iris vessels and the formation of a hyphaema. Blood collects in the anterior chamber and with the head at rest tends to gravitate downwards to form a level (Figure 10). When

Figure 9. *Corneal and scleral laceration. Cloudiness of the cornea is caused by endophthalmitis, with the anterior chamber filled with pus.*

Figure 11. *Hyphaema: blood 'stirred up' in the anterior chamber, obscuring the iris.*

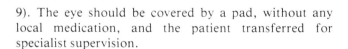

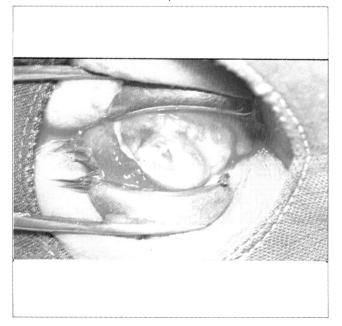

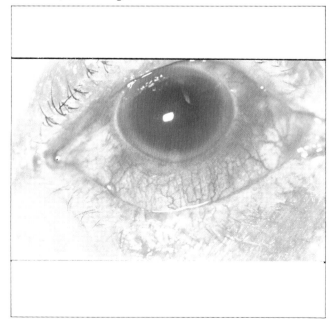

the head is moved the blood becomes distributed throughout the aqueous and obscures the details of the iris (Figure 11). Minor degrees of hyphaema occur; the red cells are then only visible with the magnification of a slit-lamp. Reabsorption of a hyphaema usually occurs within several days, but occasionally the blood persists. Red cells tend to block the normal drainage angle so that secondary glaucoma results. In this case, unless the clot is removed surgically, the cornea becomes stained with haemosiderin.

Mydriatics are not used because active dilation of the pupil can cause secondary bleeding. Once the hyphaema has been absorbed the pupil may then safely be dilated in order that a thorough examination of the peripheral retina can be made. □

Trauma to the Eye Part II

10

Traumatic Mydriasis and Iridodialysis

Damage to the constrictor muscle fibres of the iris causes a dilation of the pupil as a result of the unopposed action of the dilating fibres. This mydriasis tends to be permanent.

Tearing of the root of the iris (iridodialysis) leads to the formation of a second hole in the iris so that the patient may complain of diplopia (Figures 1 and 2). If the iridodialysis is covered by the lids it requires no treatment.

Occasionally, damage to the root of the iris causes secondary glaucoma because of the formation of scar tissue in the drainage angle. The whole of the anterior chamber appears, and is, deeper when compared with the other side, as a result of the posterior displacement of the iris.

Figure 1. *Iridodialysis: The root of the iris has been torn by a .22 air gun pellet, causing double vision.*

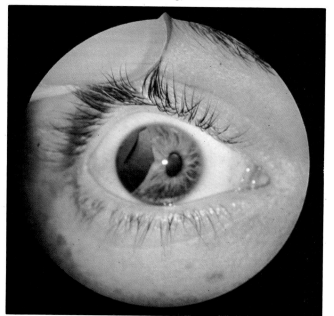

Figure 2. *Iridodialysis: the same case as in Figure 1 after surgical repair.*

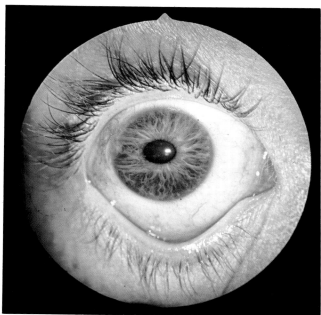

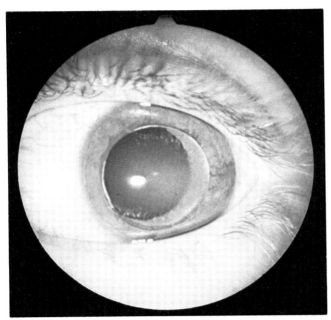

Figure 3. *Dislocation of lens: the lens displaced forward to lie in the anterior chamber in front of the iris.*

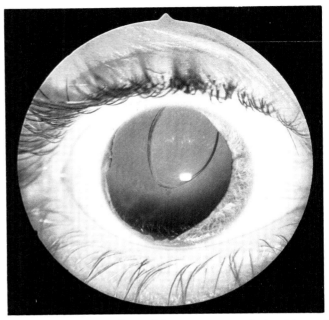

Figure 4. *Dislocation of lens: rupture of the iris and zonular fibres with posterior dislocation of the lens.*

Dislocation of the Lens and Traumatic Cataract

Dislocation of the lens occurs with a nonpenetrating type of injury to the eye. The dislocation may be forward, through the pupil, so that the lens comes to lie in the anterior chamber (Figure 3). Alternatively, the lens may be displaced backwards into the vitreous (Figure 4).

In both situations the attachment of the lens to the ciliary body by the zonular fibres is broken and all accommodation is lost. When the lens is dislocated into the vitreous, secondary glaucoma often supervenes.

A cataract can develop with relatively mild degrees of trauma. If the capsule of the lens is ruptured there is a leakage of aqueous into the lens fibres and a cataract forms. The opacity may remain localized (Figure 5) or may spread to involve the entire lens. Cataract extraction may be indicated if the visual acuity is severely affected. When the lens capsule is extensively ruptured, the lens protein is released into the aqueous and may cause severe inflammation and glaucoma. Occasionally the lens protein is totally absorbed, leaving only a thin capsule through which the patient can see when given an appropriate spectacle correction (Figure 6).

Vitreous Haemorrhage

This is usually associated with extensive injuries to the retina and choroid. The visual acuity is affected and the normal red reflex is lost over the whole or part of the fundus. The haemorrhage absorbs with complete rest in bed although large clots may tend to gravitate to the dependent part of the vitreous cavity and remain indefinitely. A thorough examination of the retina must be made to exclude the presence of a tear which could produce a retinal detachment.

Commotio Retinae

Blunt injury to the eye may produce a whitening of the retina (Figure 7). This frost-like appearance, caused by oedema, can occur at the site of the injury or may appear on the opposite side of the eye as a result of a contra-coup type of injury. When the peripheral retina is involved no permanent visual defect results, but if the oedema involves the macular area the visual acuity is often permanently reduced.

As the condition resolves the white retina becomes mottled as a result of the scattering of pigment from the pigment epithelium (Figure 8).

Retinal Detachment and Choroidal Rupture

Relatively mild trauma may cause a retinal detachment in those cases with predisposing retinal pathology. Areas of weak peripheral retina may need only a slight pull from the attached vitreous gel to develop a retinal tear and form a retinal detachment. Tears of the extreme periphery can result in a retinal dialysis. When

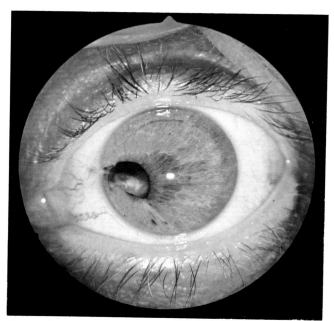

Figure 5. *Cataract: a penetrating injury at the limbus has resulted in displacement of the pupil towards the wound and a localized opacity in the lens.*

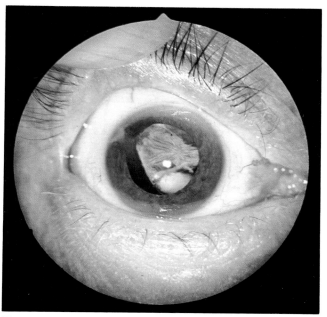

Figure 6. *Cataract: partial spontaneous reabsorption of a cataract leaving a grey capsule filling the pupillary area with a small cataract remnant above.*

the retina is torn at the ora serrata, the most anterior border of the retina, detachment of the retina ensues, but the results of surgery are excellent; normal function of the retina is restored, providing the macula was not detached.

Ruptures of the choroid occur with blunt injury and

are often associated with vitreous haemorrhage. When the fundus can be examined white crescentic tears are seen. These tears are adjacent to the disc and run parallel to its margin. When they form between the disc and macula the central vision may be impaired if there is

Figure 7. *Commotio retinae: white retinal oedema caused by a blow from a football.*

Figure 8. *Commotio retinae: the same case as in Figure 7 one year later, showing clumping of pigment over the area of affected retina.*

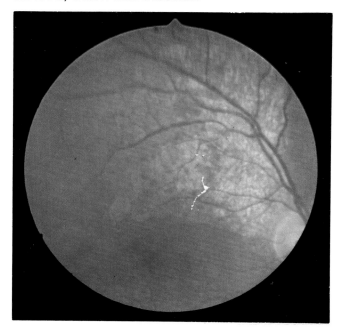

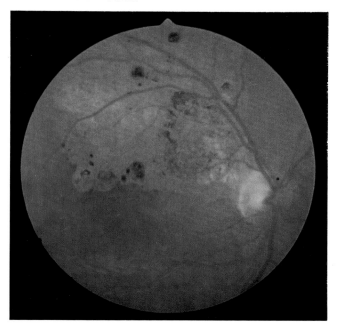

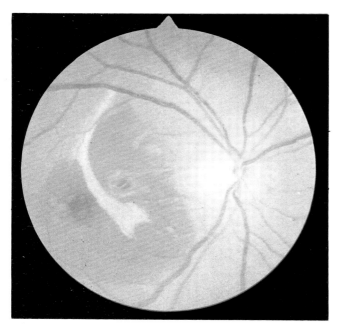

Figure 9. *Rupture of the choroid: a white crescentic break lying between the disc and macula, resulting in loss of central vision.*

associated retinal damage (Figure 9).

Optic atrophy may occur when there is damage to the blood supply of the optic nerve (Figure 10). The disc becomes pearly white with a sharp margin, in contrast to the grey disc with a blurred edge that occurs when optic atrophy follows papilloedema. The vision rapidly deteriorates and treatment is of no avail.

Penetrating Injuries

Large lacerations of the cornea or sclera are not usually missed, but penetrating injuries caused by small foreign bodies such as splinters of metal or glass may show little external damage.

Corneal wounds may be small and become plugged by iris so that the anterior chamber appears of normal depth. Damage to the lens may not become apparent for several hours, and retinal damage may not cause trouble for many weeks.

Great care should be taken if there is a history of hammering or drilling and in all cases a radiograph of the orbit should be taken.

Some foreign bodies, such as glass and plastic, are inert and may produce no reaction unless infection is also present. Iron and copper foreign bodies, however, become dispersed throughout the eye and lead to blindness if not removed.

Sympathetic Ophthalmitis

This is a form of uveitis, fortunately rare, resulting from a penetrating injury which has involved the lens and ciliary body. The inflammation which affects the

Figure 10. *Vitreous scarring: a painting of a fundus after blunt injury, with white scar tissue bands in the vitreous and pigment clumping on the retina. The white disc is caused by optic atrophy.*

Figure 11. *An eclipse burn of the macula. Note the mottled appearance of the central foveal area.*

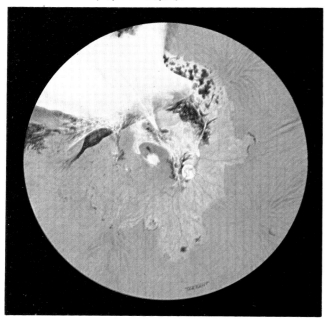

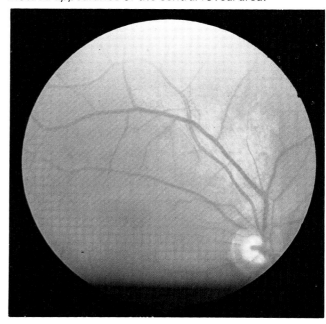

damaged eye spreads to involve the other eye after a few weeks or months. This is probably caused by an immune response which can be suppressed with systemic corticosteroids. Enucleation of a severely damaged eye within two weeks of injury will usually remove any risk to the normal eye.

Radiation Injuries

Exposure to ultraviolet light from welding apparatus (arc eye) or sunray lamps causes extreme photophobia, pain and watering of the eyes. The corneal epithelium is affected and takes up to 24 hours to heal. Treatment is analgesics, local antibiotic and padding of the eyes.

Infrared radiation penetrates the eye and is absorbed by the lens, causing a cataract typically seen in glassblowers.

Burns of the retina are occasionally found in patients working with laser equipment. The macula may suffer an eclipse burn if the sun is observed without adequate protection. The damage produced is irreversible and central vision is permanently defective (Figure 11).   □

Cataract

11

A cataract is an opacity in the lens, and is associated with an increased water content. The normally transparent soluble protein of the lens becomes insoluble and opaque. This change occurs in the elderly so that after the age of 65 years some degree of cataract is found in most patients. However, developmental factors, inflammation, trauma and systemic disease may also cause cataracts.

Types of Cataract

Congenital

Several types of congenital cataract have been described, of differing appearance and position in the lens (Figure 1). The lamellar cataract accounts for nearly half of all congenital cataracts and is important because it lies on the visual axis (Figure 2). When the pupil is dilated a disc-like opacity is visible, around which is a rim of clear lens. There may be projections from the surface radiating like spokes of a wheel.

Congenital cataracts are most commonly seen as a complication of maternal rubella, but they may also occur with defective calcium metabolism.

Senile

There are two types of senile cataract:

1. Nuclear sclerosis in which the centre of the lens becomes optically more dense. The colour in the early stages may be yellow or orange and later can change to dark brown (Figure 3). This colour change can produce marked alteration in perceived colour values. As the change is gradual it may not be noted by the patient until the cataract is removed and the true colours are seen again.

2. Cortical opacities which occur as peripheral spokes pointing at the centre of the pupil, or as opacities

Figure 1. *Anterior polar cataract: a localized opacity on the anterior surface of the lens, usually bilateral, nonprogressive and not affecting the vision.*

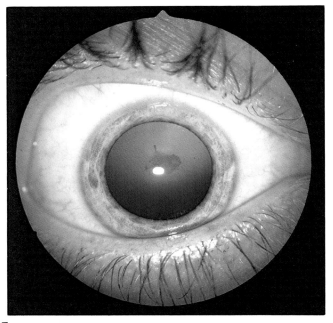

77

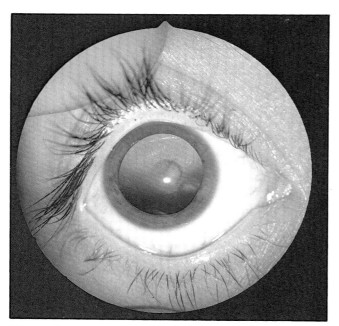

Figure 2. *Lamellar cataract: a central disc-like opacity which, when dense, produces marked visual deterioration because of its position on the visual axis. It is usually bilateral.*

beneath the posterior capsule of the lens (Figures 4 and 5). Both can be seen with the ophthalmoscope, in silhouette against the red reflex of the fundus (Figures 6 and 7).

Figure 3. *Nuclear sclerosis: a dark brown cataract in the late stages.*

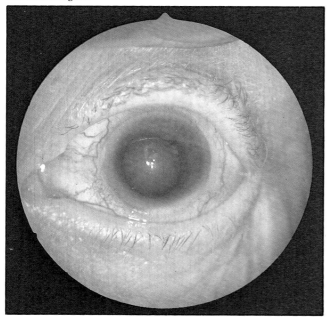

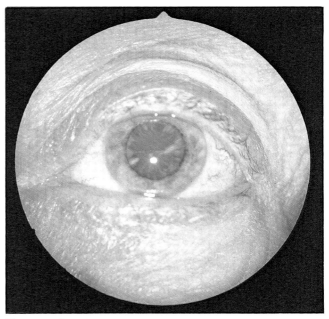

Figure 4. *Cortical cataract: radiating spoke-like opacities affecting the peripheral lens with a few extensions towards the centre. Visual acuity may be good until central opacities develop.*

Cortical cataracts are associated with hydration and swelling of the lens (Figure 8). When the entire lens is opaque the cataract is described as mature (Figure 9). If a mature cataract is not removed it may progress to the stage of hypermaturity, when lens protein escaping through the capsule causes severe intraocular inflammatory changes.

Symptoms

A painless gradual deterioration in vision is the commonest presenting symptom. The vision varies with the lighting, often being worse in bright light and better when dark glasses are worn. When the cataract affects the peripheral part of the lens the visual loss is not as severe as that caused by an opacity on the visual axis.

The development of nuclear sclerosis produces myopia, so that a patient who previously needed reading glasses finds that he manages better without them—a slight compensation for the developing cataract.

Nuclear sclerosis may also produce double vision as a result of the dense central portion of the lens acting as a stronger lens than the peripheral part. This diplopia is uniocular, unlike that associated with a squint of recent onset which disappears when one eye is shut.

Haloes and stars are commonly seen around lights because of the diffraction of light. These whitish yellow haloes usually differ from those caused by glaucoma,

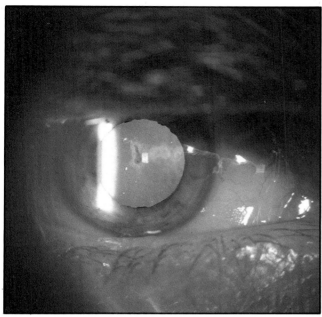

Figure 5. *Cortical cataract: a comma-shaped opacity appearing on the visual axis beneath the posterior capsule. Vision is impaired in the early stages.*

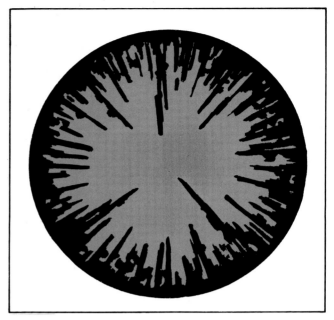

Figure 6. *Cortical cataract: silhouette of spoke opacities.*

which are typically rainbow coloured. Spots or opacities in the visual field may be seen. These move as the eye moves and are more noticeable against a light background.

Treatment

There is no medical treatment for cataract. Surgical removal of the lens should be performed at a time that is suited to the visual demands of the patient. Some elderly patients are content with 6/24 vision, while a young draughtsman may be severely incapacitated with a level of 6/12. The popular belief that the patient must wait until the cataract is 'ripe' is incorrect.

Inpatient treatment for a routine operation lasts about one week. Surgery can be performed under local or general anaesthesia although in the United Kingdom the majority of cases receive a general anaesthetic. The patient is mobilized the day after the operation. The eye is kept padded for the first few days, after which dark glasses or temporary aphakic glasses are worn. The latter contain an approximate lens and give some vision until the final glasses are ordered six weeks after surgery. Depending on their vision, patients can usually return to work in six weeks if their job is sedentary, or slightly longer if they are involved in particularly strenuous activities.

Unilateral cataract is the cause of much misun-

derstanding. After operation the aphakic eye is markedly hypermetropic and clear vision can only be obtained when this is corrected. The use of glasses produces a magnifying effect so that the image seen is one-third larger than normal. Therefore, correction with glasses is only possible if the patient accepts that he

Figure 7. *Cortical cataract: silhouette of posterior subcapsular opacities.*

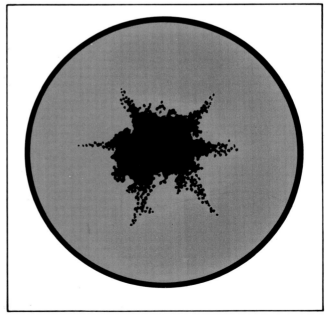

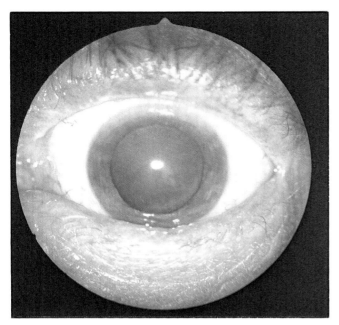

Figure 8. *Cortical cataract: immature cataract not completely opaque, with a slight red reflex visible.*

will see with one eye. If he is willing and able to wear a contact lens in the operated eye it is then possible to use the two eyes together.

Methods of Extraction

There are two methods of lens extraction:

Figure 9. *Mature cataract: completely opaque swollen lens.*

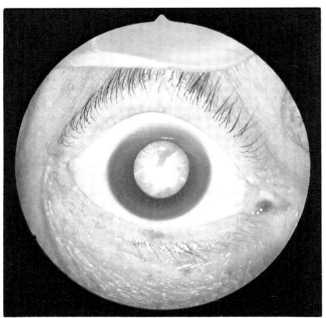

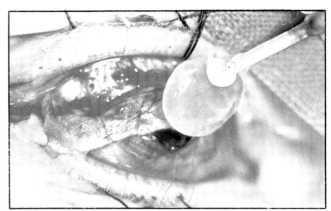

Figure 10. *Intracapsular cataract extraction: the lens, with nuclear sclerosis, is adherent to the cryoprobe.*

1. Intracapsular: the cataractous lens complete with its capsule is removed with the cryoprobe (a freezing probe that adheres to the lens) (Figure 10). This is the commonest operation for cataract.

2. Extracapsular: in a patient under the age of 30 years, removal of the capsule by rupture of the zonular fibres usually predisposes to retinal detachment. The capsule is, therefore, incised and the lens contents are aspirated. Several instruments are available for this technique, which has the advantage of a small entry wound into the eye and, therefore, a short hospital stay.

Correction of Aphakia

Glasses

This is the commonest method for correcting the hypermetropia of aphakia, but it has limitations. In addition to the magnification effect already mentioned there are considerable distortions with the high power convex lenses. An undistorted image is only achieved when the centre of the lens is used. Even then, horizontal lines may appear to bend at the end and verticals, such as door posts, to curve inwards. The inability to accommodate interferes with the assessment of distance, so that simple tasks such as pouring a cup of tea are at first difficult to perform. With perseverence, however, these complications are usually overcome within a matter of weeks.

Contact Lenses

Hard or soft contact lenses may be used in aphakia. The distortions are less than those with glasses, but are replaced by other complications. Many patients are of an age when their manual dexterity is deteriorating and they cannot manage the insertion and removal of the lens. In the younger age group, however, the results with contact lenses are excellent.

Intraocular Implant

Plastic lenses can be inserted into the eye at the time of the removal of the cataract. These lenses lie either in the pupil or just behind it, so that they replace the cataractous lens. Only the distance vision is corrected, as the patient is still unable to accommodate, and reading glasses are required. However, there are many complications to be overcome with this method, the worst being corneal oedema, before it can become a safe routine procedure. ☐

Glaucoma

12

Glaucoma is a term used to describe a number of conditions which are characterized by raised intraocular pressure, cupping of the optic disc and visual field defects. The pathology lies at the optic nerve head which becomes ischaemic as a result of an imbalance between the intraocular pressure and the perfusion pressure in the capillaries of the disc.

The normal intraocular pressure, 15 to 20 mm Hg, is maintained by a balance of the production of the aqueous and its drainage from the eye. The aqueous produced by the ciliary body epithelium passes through the pupil, and leaves the anterior chamber by draining through the trabecular meshwork in the angle into the canal of Schlemm, and thence to the episcleral veins (Figure 1). Glaucoma is caused by an obstruction at the level of the trabecular meshwork.

The different types of glaucoma can be grouped as follows:

1. Open angle glaucoma or chronic simple glaucoma.
2. Narrow angle glaucoma.
3. Congenital glaucoma.
4. Secondary glaucoma.

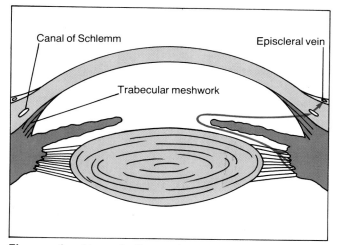

Figure 1. *Normal flow of aqueous. Aqueous is produced by the ciliary body epithelium; it passes through the pupil and leaves the eye through the trabecular meshwork, Schlemm's canal and the episcleral veins.*

first-degree relatives over the age of 40 are likely to have the condition.

Presentation

The diagnosis may be very difficult as the patient may be completely free of symptoms, with the eye gradually adapting to the insidious rise of pressure. The first presentation may be during routine refraction when cupping of the disc is noticed. Occasionally, some blurring of vision with difficulty in reading is experienced, but headaches and eye ache are rare. The

Open Angle or Chronic Simple Glaucoma

This is the commonest form of glaucoma in those over 40 years of age, and is divided equally between the sexes. There is a strong hereditary element, so the investigation of both siblings and children of affected patients should be considered. Ten per cent of these

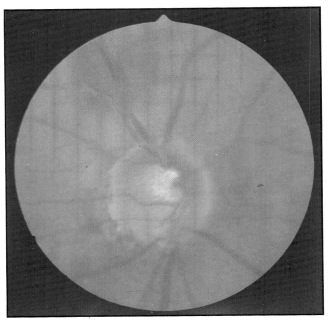

Figure 2. *Disc cupping: the lower border of the cup is enlarged to give an upper half visual field defect.*

sclera is white with a bright clear cornea and active pupil. The anterior chamber is of normal depth. It is possible to examine the width of the angle of the anterior chamber using a gonioscope—a special type of contact lens.

Figure 3. *Disc cupping: both upper and lower borders of the disc are cupped with nasal displacement of the vessels.*

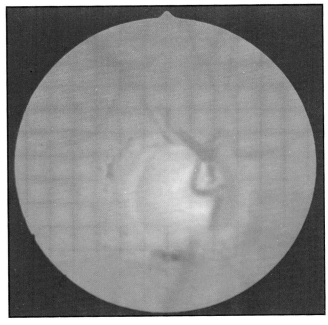

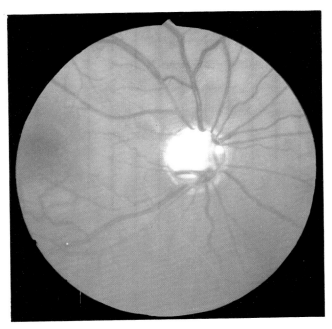

Figure 4. *Disc cupping: advanced case with the vessels disappearing over the edge of the cupped disc.*

Ophthalmoscopic Changes

These are the most obvious feature. The disc may have a white atrophic halo around it with haemorrhages on the disc margin. The central physiological cup becomes enlarged, usually at the upper and lower borders, forming a vertical oval (Figures 2 and 3). The vessels become displaced nasally, and are seen to loop over the edge of the cup to reappear on its floor (Figure 4). The atrophic white cupped area gradually enlarges until it occupies almost the entire area of the disc.

Visual Field Defects

These defects are characteristic (Figures 5 to 8). They start as isolated scotomata (blind areas) extending in an arc above and below fixation to join up with the blind spot (the arcuate scotoma). These field defects gradually enlarge to become continuous with the peripheral field loss that occurs on the nasal side (nasal step). In the untreated patient there is an inevitable progression until only a small area of vision may be left in the centre. With this the patient may still have a good level of visual acuity despite the severe overall loss of visual field.

Intraocular Pressure

Accurate assessment of intraocular pressure can only be made by applanation tonometry. Digital assessment is only very approximate. The level of intraocular pressure

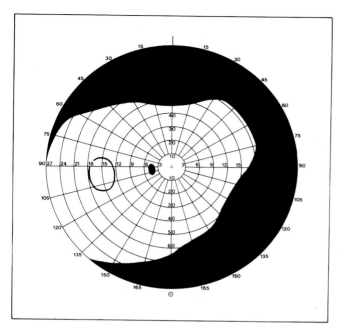

Figure 5. *Normal left field of vision: peripheral and central field of left eye showing normal smaller nasal field due to the nose and the normal blind spot.*

can vary considerably, but levels above 25 mm Hg must be regarded with suspicion. Occasionally, levels above normal are found without any field defects having developed. This is ocular hypertension and should be watched carefully as it may progress and develop the

Figure 6. *Glaucomatous field defects: an area of visual loss extending from the blind spot (arcuate scotoma), and loss of the upper nasal field (nasal step).*

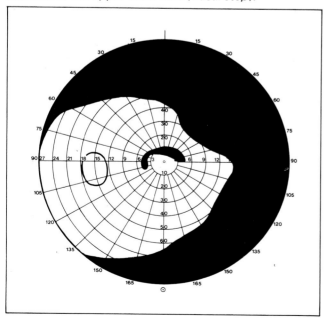

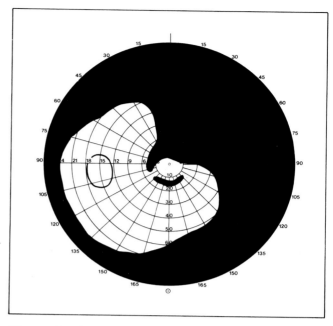

Figure 7. *Glaucomatous field defects: the upper arcuate scotoma has linked with the nasal step. A lower arcuate scotoma has appeared.*

typical disc cupping and field defects of chronic simple glaucoma.

Treatment

Treatment is always initially medical and only when this

Figure 8. *Glaucomatous field defects: loss of all the field of vision except for two small areas in an untreated case of chronic simple glaucoma.*

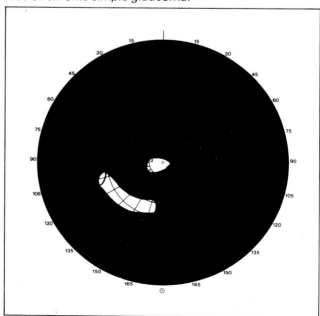

has failed is surgery considered. The success of treatment is gauged not only by the fall in intraocular pressure, but also by the prevention of further field loss. The intraocular pressure shows a diurnal variation, with the highest pressure in the waking hours of the morning. Successful treatment must control this rise and keep an even level throughout the twenty-four hours.

Local Administration

Pilocarpine. Despite the advent of numerous drugs, pilocarpine remains the drug of choice. It is a cholinergic agent and is administered by drops at six-hourly intervals in strengths of one to four per cent. It probably acts by increasing the outflow of aqueous. It also causes miosis, reducing the light entering the eye. This, together with a small degree of central or axial cataract, can markedly lower the visual acuity. In young patients pilocarpine may cause blurring of vision for one to one and a half hours after instillation, because of its effect on the ciliary muscle.

Pilocarpine can also be administered by means of Ocuserts, whereby a continuous release of the drug is achieved from a small plastic pledget retained under the upper or lower lids. In some cases this produces a better control of intraocular pressure, without the repeated instillation of drops. The blurring of vision noted after drop therapy is also improved.

Adrenaline. This is administered as one half or one per cent drops. The lowering of the intraocular pressure is achieved by reduction of the secretion of aqueous and by increasing the drainage from the eye. As adrenaline dilates the pupil it should not be given if the anterior chamber is shallow, in case closure of the angle occurs (Figure 9).

Guanethidine may also be used in conjunction with adrenaline, whose action it potentiates. However, both adrenaline and guanethidine tend to make the eyes red and irritable.

Timolol is a recent addition to the topical drugs and is proving very successful. A beta adrenergic blocking agent, it acts by reducing aqueous secretion. It is used in strengths of 0.25 and 0.5 per cent, given every 12 hours and is free of the visual and hyperaemic complications of other glaucoma therapy.

Carbochol, eserine and phospholine iodide all produce a lowering of intraocular pressure but, due to side-effects, are not commonly used.

Systemic Administration

Local therapy can be aided by the systemic use of acetazolamide (Diamox 250 mg up to four times a day) and dichlorphenamide (Daranide 50 mg up to four times a day). Both diminish aqueous secretion, but have unpleasant side-effects. Tingling in the hands and feet,

Figure 9. *Melanin deposits: long-term adrenaline treatment may cause harmless black deposits in the conjunctiva.*

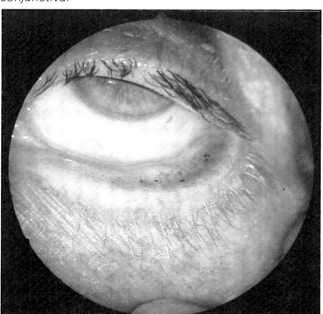

Figure 10. *Glaucoma drainage operation: shows a small bleb of conjunctiva at 12 o'clock into which aqueous drains.*

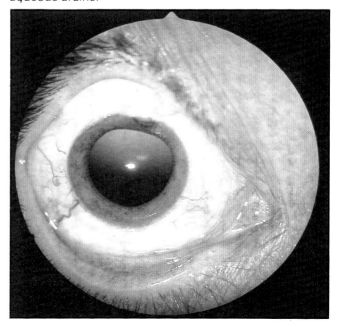

indigestion, renal calculi and occasionally skin rashes and blood dyscrasias can occur.

Surgical Treatment

Medical treatment may fail because of inadequate pressure control, failure by the patient to maintain medication or because of drug side-effects. Surgical methods aim to provide an alternative drainage channel for aqueous from inside the eye to the subconjunctival space (Figure 10).

Trabeculectomy is now the standard drainage operation and involves the removal of a segment of sclera involving the canal of Schlemm and the trabecular meshwork.

Narrow Angle Glaucoma

This occurs in middle-age and is twice as common in women. It is commoner in the hypermetropic eye, which is shorter in length and has a shallower anterior chamber (Figure 11).

Presentation

Subacute Attacks

These may be confused with migraine. Partial closure of the angle can occur when the pupil is semidilated, and the contact between the iris and lens prevents the normal flow of aqueous through the pupil. The increasing pressure behind the iris causes it to balloon

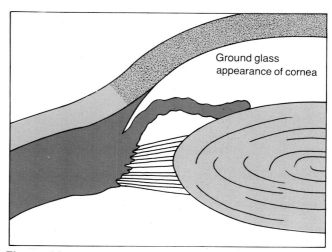

Figure 12. *Narrow angle glaucoma: the semidilated iris is ballooned forwards by the aqueous, so closing the angle. The cornea becomes waterlogged because of the increased intraocular pressure.*

forwards, so blocking the angle (Figure 12). The increased intraocular pressure forces fluid into the cornea, which causes the typical appearance of 'haloes'. These are seen around lights as coloured rings. The attacks, which usually occur in the evenings, resolve during the night due to the pupillary constriction that occurs with sleep. Mild attacks may occur for several months before the development of an acute attack.

Acute Attacks

The acute attack has a dramatic presentation. The patient complains of intense pain in and around the eye, and its severity may lead to marked shock with vomiting. This can result in wasting valuable time while a gastrointestinal cause is sought. The eye is red with dilation of the conjunctival vessels over the whole of the sclera, in contrast to the limited redness adjacent to the limbus in uveitis (Figure 13).

The cornea is hazy, obscuring the details of the iris. The anterior chamber is shallow, so that the surface of the iris is convex and appears to line the inside of the cornea. The pupil is typically nonreacting, semidilated and vertically oval. The iris appears muddy with a spiral effect of the stroma.

The intraocular pressue is markedly raised and the eye feels stony hard when compared with the other eye by digital palpation.

Treatment

Immediate action is required if the vision is to be saved. Miotics are used, to constrict the pupil and relieve the

Figure 11. *Narrow and open angles: (a) the narrow angle between the iris and the cornea found in the small hypermetropic eye with a large lens and a shallow anterior chamber and (b) the open angle of the normal eye.*

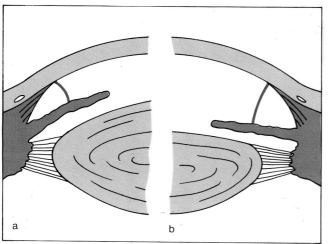

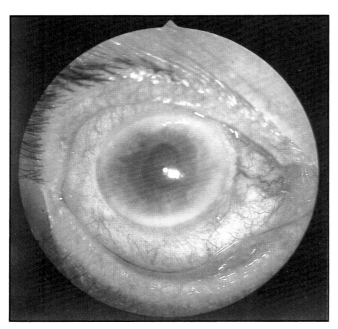

Figure 13. *Acute narrow angle glaucoma: the typical red eye with a hazy cornea and a fixed and vertically oval pupil.*

blockage of the angle by the iris. Intensive treatment with four per cent Pilocarpine drops every five minutes for half an hour together with intramuscular acetazolamide 500 mg will usually lower the pressure if the attack has been present for only a few hours. Additional treatment can be given with osmotic agents—oral glycerol, a sickly unpalatable drink, or intravenous mannitol. If the pressure is not lowered in 24 to 36 hours, permanent visual damage is inevitable. It is very important to constrict the fellow eye as it is not uncommon for the condition to occur bilaterally. Surgical treatment by means of a drainage operation is indicated if the pressure cannot be controlled by medical therapy.

If the acute attack is satisfactorily contained a peripheral iridectomy is performed. This allows aqueous to pass through the iris into the angle and so breaks the sequence of events normally leading to an angle closure attack. Prophylactic iridectomy should also be carried out on the other eye; although it may be unaffected, it is at risk.

Congenital Glaucoma

This form of glaucoma, also called buphthalmos, usually presents in the first three months of life. It is most commonly bilateral and affects males more often than females. It is caused by an abnormality in the development of the angle of the anterior chamber, preventing normal drainage of aqueous.

The raised intraocular pressure results in the enlargement of the eyeball, with the diameter of the cornea also enlarged (Figure 14). The cornea may become oedematous and cloudy and the anterior chamber is deepened. The most striking features of the condition are photophobia, blepharospasm (inability to open the eyes) and epiphora.

Surgical treatment is essential if the sight is to be saved. Goniotomy is performed to divide any abnormal tissue covering the trabecular meshwork. The best results are obtained in those cases operated on before the age of three months, but even then several operations may be necessary.

Secondary Glaucoma

A secondary rise in intraocular pressure occurs as a result of poor drainage of aqueous from the eye. This most commonly occurs when the trabecular meshwork is obstructed. This can occur in iritis when protein and white cells are released into the anterior chamber. A similar blockage occurs with red cells when trauma to the eye causes a hyphaema, or when lens protein leaks from a hypermature cataract.

In pigmentary glaucoma the angle becomes heavily pigmented due to the dispersion of pigment from the iris, while in pseudoexfoliation of the lens there is a white deposit in the angle causing a rise in pressure.

Figure 14. *Congenital glaucoma: the enlarged hazy cornea of an eye with marked photophobia, blepharospasm and epiphora.*

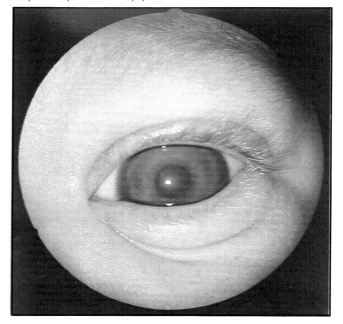

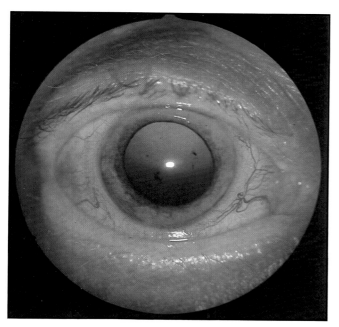

Figure 15. *Thrombotic glaucoma: neovascularization of the iris (rubeosis iridis) following central retinal vein occlusion. A similar picture can occur with diabetes.*

In diabetes and following obstruction of the central retinal vein, neovascularization of the iris (rubeosis iridis) extends into the angle to block the trabecular meshwork (Figure 15).

Glaucoma may also result from scarring of the trabecular meshwork following blunt injury to the eye. The iris and lens are pushed backwards so that recession of the angle occurs, with deepening of the anterior chamber.

A chronic form of glaucoma can be produced in certain susceptible patients by the use of local steroid preparations. The stronger preparations betamethasone (Betnesol) and dexamethasone (Maxidex) can produce a clinical picture similar to chronic simple glaucoma after only a few weeks. These drugs should, therefore, only be used under the guidance of an ophthalmic department.

Squint

13

There are many different terms used in the English language to describe a squint—for example, strabismus, cast, turn, wall-eyed and cross-eyed—but they may mean different things to different people. Even the term squint may be used to describe the screwing up of the eyes.

A squint is present when the axes of the two eyes are differently aligned. One eye (the fixing eye) will look at an object while the other (the squinting eye) is directed elsewhere, so that normal binocular vision is impossible.

Amblyopia and Double Vision

In young children a squint results in the suppression by the brain of the image from the squinting eye in order to prevent double vision. If this suppression is not corrected it will progress to amblyopia (lazy eye). After the age of eight years treatment for amblyopia is usually ineffective and the reduction in vision is permanent, but referral is still advised.

When an adult with normal binocular vision develops a squint, double vision is produced. This is because the brain is unable to suppress the image from the squinting eye.

Causes of Squints

Squints are produced by motor, sensory or central defects. Sensory defects are caused by poor vision, for which ptosis of the lid, corneal scarring, congenital cataract or macular malfunction are responsible, while central defects are the result of brain damage. Sensory and central defects both produce nonparalytic or concomitant squints. Motor defects such as ocular muscle paresis will cause an abnormal movement of the eye producing a paralytic squint.

Nonparalytic or Concomitant Squint

This is the commonest type of squint and is typically seen in children.

History and Presentation

There is often a strong family history of squints. The child is usually brought for attention because of the

Figure 1. *Right convergent squint. Displacement of the corneal light reflex to the temporal side of the right pupil is shown.*

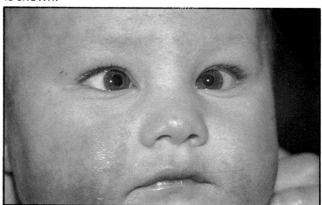

91

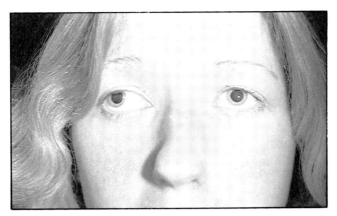

Figure 2. *Right divergent squint. Displacement nasally of the right corneal light reflex is shown.*

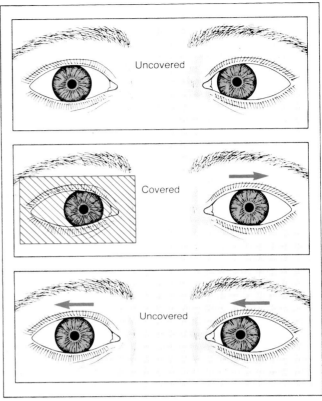

Figure 3. *Left convergent squint. Movements of the eyes with the cover test are shown.*

appearance of the eyes rather than for double vision, although small-angled squints may pass unnoticed until the child is old enough for a visual acuity test, when a lazy eye is detected.

Examination

The squint is present wherever the eyes are turned and the angle of the squint is constant. It is usually horizontal and may be either convergent (inwards) or divergent (outwards). It is rarely vertical.

When the eye is convergent the reflection of a light is seen displaced temporally and more sclera is visible on the temporal side of the cornea (Figure 1). With a divergent squint the findings are reversed (Figure 2).

The Cover Test

The cover test is used to confirm the presence of a squint. With a light held at a third of a metre from the patient, one eye is covered while the opposite eye is watched for movement. Figure 3 shows a left convergent squint. On covering the left eye no movement is detected as the straight right eye is already looking at the light. When the right eye is covered the left eye moves outwards. When the right eye is uncovered both eyes move so that the right becomes straight and the left convergent.

Figure 4 shows an alternating convergent squint. Initially, the convergent left eye will move when the right eye is covered. On uncovering the right eye there is no movement of the left eye and the right eye is seen to be convergent. This occurs because the patient has no preference to look with his right or left eye.

Figure 5 shows the movements with the cover test for a left divergent squint.

Visual Acuity

Accurate assessment of the visual acuity in children under the age of two years is difficult. A refraction is carried out using a cycloplegic and mydriatic drug such as atropine to prevent the child accommodating and giving the false impression of myopia. Spectacles may then be prescribed if there is any obvious refractive error.

The fundi are examined while the pupils are dilated for a refraction, so that any ocular abnormality can be excluded.

In the older but still illiterate age group the Sheridan Gardiner Test is used, in which the child matches a set of letters to differing single letters held at a distance by the examiner (Figure 6). Although this test is in common use, its results are sometimes open to suspicion.

Management

The aim of successful treatment is to produce equal visual acuity in each eye with good binocular vision, and to this end no child is too young to refer for examination.

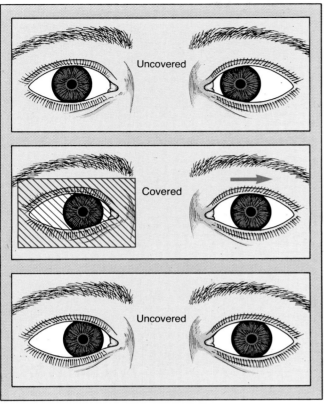

Figure 4. *Alternating convergent squint. Movements of the convergent eye with the cover test are shown.*

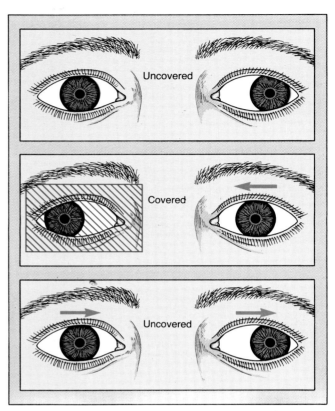

Figure 5. *Left divergent squint. Movements of the eyes with the cover test are shown.*

Figure 6. *Sheridan Gardiner Test. This is used to test visual acuity in the three- to five-year-old age group.*

Spectacles

Spectacles will be required to correct any significant refractive error.

The eye of the newborn child is only three-quarters of the adult size, resulting in hypermetropia. This means that to see clearly at a distance the child must accommodate, and to see close objects even more accommodative effort is required. As there is a close link between the effort needed to accommodate and to converge to see a near object, then the over-focussing of hypermetropia can be accompanied by over-convergence. Therefore, the child has a convergent squint when looking at close objects. This type of squint is called an accommodative squint and may be controlled with glasses (Figures 7 and 8).

Occasionally, bifocal lenses may be used in accommodative squints for a short period.

Occlusion

Occlusion is carried out to improve the vision in an amblyopic eye to match that of the normal eye. The normal eye is covered either by sticking plaster directly

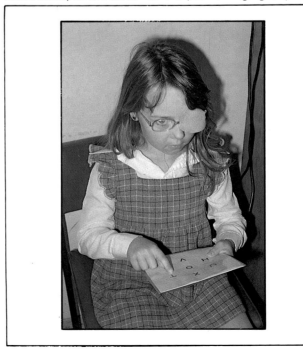

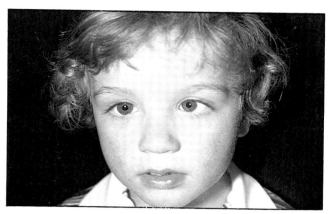

Figure 7. *Left convergent squint (accommodative squint).*

Figure 8. *Left convergent squint (accommodative squint) controlled with glasses.*

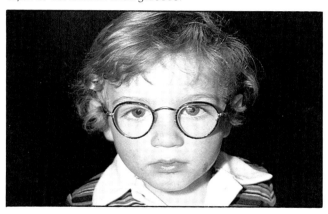

on the face (Figure 9), or on to the glasses if they are worn. It should be used continuously for varying lengths of time each day, under the close supervision of an orthoptic department.

Drops

The accommodative type of squint may respond to ecothiopate drops (Phospholine iodide). However, prolonged use is not advisable as cataracts can be produced and the suppression of serum pseudocholinesterase makes the use of succinylcholine in general anaesthesia hazardous.

Surgery

Surgical correction of a squint is necessary when the preceding methods have either partially or totally failed to control it. The method involves weakening by recession and strengthening by resection of the affected muscles.

If squint surgery can be performed within the first few months of life the prognosis for binocular vision is improved. In approximately 30 per cent of cases a second operation is required. One relatively common postoperative complication is the formation of a granuloma over the site of the resected muscle (Figure 10). This responds well to a local corticosteroid preparation.

Paralytic Squint

This type of squint is most commonly seen in adults who have already developed normal binocular vision.

Presentation

The onset is usually sudden and is marked by double vision. There are three main findings:

1. Abnormal position of the eyes.
2. Limitation of movement of the affected eye.
3. Abnormal head posture.

From Figure 11 it can be seen that paralysis of the right medial rectus will result in the eye becoming divergent

Figure 9. *Occlusion. Sticking plaster is used to cover the normal eye in the treatment of amblyopia.*

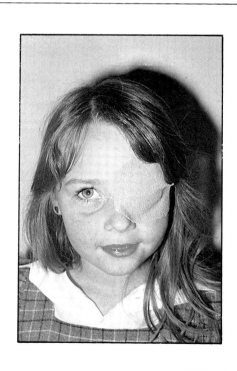

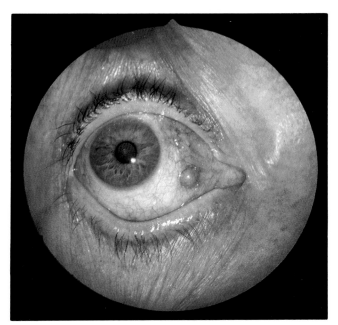

Figure 10. *Granuloma: swelling over the lower end of the resected medial rectus muscle.*

due to the unopposed action of the right lateral rectus (Figure 12). When the right eye movements are tested, no movement towards the nose is possible beyond the midline position.

The double vision is worse when looking to the left, i.e. in the direction of the action of the affected muscle, and least when looking to the right. The patient, therefore, tends to turn her head to the left so that the eyes are kept in the least troublesome position. So for horizontal muscles the abnormal head position is to turn the head towards the side of the affected muscle.

Vertical muscle palsies produce more complicated findings in which the head may be turned and tilted to try to minimize the diplopia.

Causes

The palsy may be due to a lesion either in the muscle or in its nerve supply.

Muscular weakness can be associated with endocrine exophthalmos and myasthenia gravis.

Lesions in the nerve supply are seen in association with diabetes and hypertension and are probably the result of interference with the vascular supply to the nerve. The third cranial nerve is most commonly affected, although isolated sixth-nerve palsy can occur. Aneurysms of the intracranial arteries and tumours, including metastases, are less likely causes.

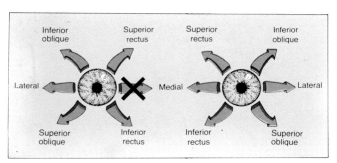

Figure 11. *Actions of eye muscles, illustrating the effect of paralysis of the right medial rectus.*

In the under-40 age group multiple sclerosis is a common cause of cranial nerve lesions. Palsy of the fourth cranial nerve is nearly always the result of trauma.

Management

Investigation for the underlying cause of a paralytic squint is the primary concern. Symptomatic treatment to relieve the diplopia is by occlusion of the squinting eye or occasionally by a prismatic spectacle correction.

Surgical treatment is never considered before six months and only then if tests show that the angle of the squint is static.

Latent Squint

This type of squint occurs in those patients whose eyes are normally kept straight by good binocular vision. When the eye muscles are fatigued, the effort of keeping the eyes correctly aligned is too great and one eye tends to wander. This is a latent squint. If the deviation of the

Figure 12. *Right divergent squint. Paralysis of the right medial rectus has resulted in a divergent squint because of the unopposed action of the lateral rectus.*

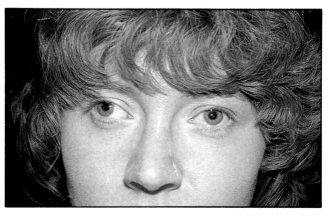

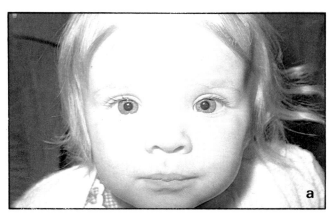

Figure 13a. *Epicanthus. There is no squint when the child is looking straight ahead.*

eye becomes constant, the squint is termed a manifest squint. The term phoria is also used to describe a latent squint with esophoria being convergent and exophoria being divergent.

Surgery is occasionally required to strengthen the muscles.

Pseudosquint and Epicanthus

This is due to a facial abnormality: the bridge of the nose is wider than normal and an epicanthic fold may be present. The latter is a bilateral fold of skin connecting the medial end of the upper and lower lids.

Figure 13a shows a typical case where no squint is visible when the child looks straight ahead. On looking to the left (Figure 13b) the right eye seems to turn in more than the left eye turns out. The reverse situation occurs on looking to the right, when the left eye appears to over-converge (Figure 13c). Because the facial changes may mask a true squint, referral of these cases is necessary. ☐

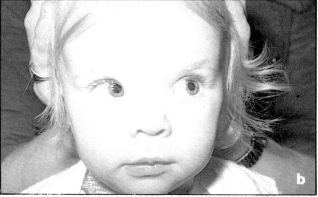

Figure 13b. *Epicanthus. There is an apparent right convergent squint when looking to the left.*

Figure 13c. *Epicanthus. There is an apparent left convergent squint when looking to the right.*

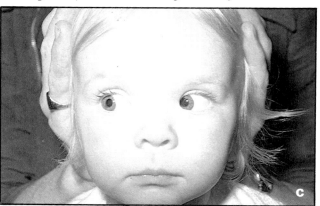

Congenital Deformities

14

The commonest congenital defects affecting the lens, extraocular muscles and the anterior chamber have already been discussed under the headings of cataract, squint and glaucoma. There remain some less common anomalies whose appearance may be confused with other conditions, and others that deserve mention in their own right.

Facial Deformities

Sturge-Weber Syndrome

This consists of facial angioma, chronic glaucoma and meningeal angioma. The obvious facial lesion (naevus flammeus) usually involves only half the face and follows the distribution of the fifth cranial nerve (Figure 1). The lips may show hypertrophy, and eyelid anomalies are usually associated with ocular involvement. Haemangiomata of the conjunctiva and the choroid are common and are associated with chronic glaucoma. Retinal detachment and cataract may develop, for which treatment is usually unsuccessful. The intracranial lesion is an angioma overlying the parietal and occipital lobes. The resulting pressure atrophy may lead to mental deterioration, fits and hemiparesis. Skull x-ray shows calcification of the cerebral cortex with a double contour-line marking.

Hypertelorism

This condition may be confused with epicanthus. There is a wide displacement of the orbits with a broadening of the bridge of the nose (Figure 2). Epicanthic folds may be present, and a divergent squint and optic atrophy may also occur. The condition is rare.

Ptosis

Ptosis is characterized by a drooping of the upper lid (Figure 3). It is most commonly unilateral and may be associated with weakness of the superior rectus muscle. There is often a strong hereditary tendency. If the lid covers the pupil, early treatment of the condition is indicated to avert the risk of amblyopia. If the condition

Figure 1. *Sturge-Weber syndrome: facial haemangioma with hypertrophy of lip and involvement of the eye with cataract formation.*

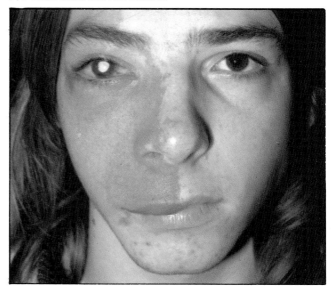

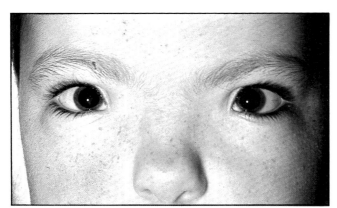

Figure 2. *Hypertelorism: displacement of orbits with wide bridge of the nose.*

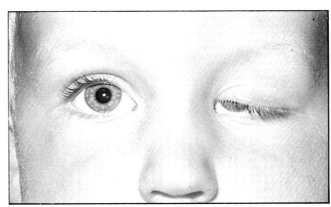

Figure 3. *Ptosis, showing some residual action of the levator muscle due to the presence of a palpebral crease in the upper lid.*

is bilateral, the child may adopt an abnormal posture with the head tilted back in order to see below the drooping lids.

When the pupil is not covered, surgery may safely be postponed until the age of three or four years. Shortening of the levator muscle is effective providing the muscle is not paralysed. If there is no action of the levator palpebrae superioris the usual palpebral crease in the upper lid is missing. A sling operation, using a strip of fascia lata, lifts the lid by attaching it to the frontalis muscle.

Dermoid Cysts

These inclusion cysts are relatively common around the eyes, and are seen in the outer third of the upper lid (Figure 4). The skin is freely mobile over the firm rounded cyst, which may be adherent to the underlying bone. Occasionally, it extends into the orbit.

Surgical excision is usually indicated for cosmetic reasons as these cysts tend gradually to increase in size.

Dermoid cyst of the cornea is a raised, pinkish swelling, sometimes pigmented and hairy (Figure 5). Removal of the lesion is necessary not only for cosmetic reasons, but also because of the gradual encroachment on to the cornea.

Coloboma

The term coloboma is used to describe a condition in which there is a defect in the normal anatomy of the eye. Structures that can be involved include the iris, ciliary body, retina, choroid and disc. The fault lies in incomplete closure of the embryonic tissue through which the vascular supply reaches the developing eye and the nerve fibres from the retina leave it.

When the iris and ciliary body are involved the defect

Figure 4. *Dermoid cyst: smooth, rounded swelling above the lateral canthus.*

Figure 5. *Dermoid cyst: limbal dermoid with surface pigmentation and hairs.*

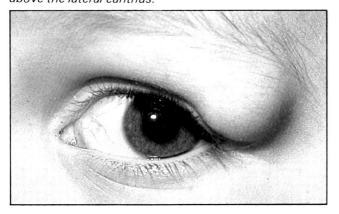

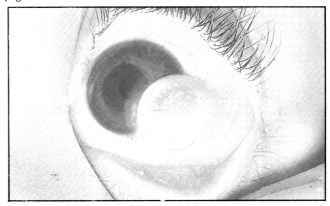

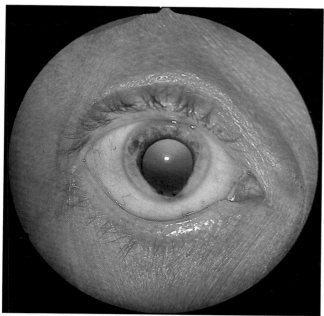

Figure 6. *Coloboma of iris: typical inferior notching of the iris.*

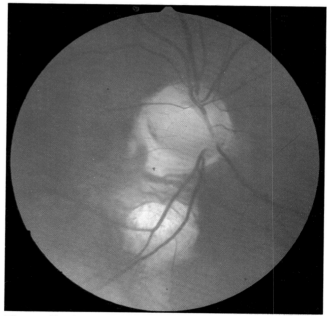

Figure 7. *Coloboma of choroid and retina: defective area of choroid and retina extending to the edge of the disc with bare sclera visible.*

is usually positioned downwards and inwards (Figure 6). The iris has a notch extending back into the ciliary body so that the pupil becomes oval or pear-shaped.

With coloboma of the retina and choroid the lesion is in the lower half of the eye and varies in size. The white sclera is visible where the overlying retina and choroid are absent (Figure 7). The defect may be continuous with the disc or isolated from it. It may be confused with old inactive choroiditis, but the inflammatory lesion is associated with more pigmentary changes around the edge than the coloboma.

Involvement of the disc by the coloboma may be only slight or it may include the entire disc with considerable distortion of its normal shape (Figure 8).

The visual acuity is usually affected in those cases where there are large defects in the fundus.

Figure 8. *Coloboma of disc: grossly distorted disc is surrounded by white sclera with complete absence of choroid and retina. (Fellow eye of patient in Figure 7).*

Aniridia

In this hereditary condition the iris appears to be totally absent. The whole lens and zonule are visible (Figure 9), and the rudimentary iris may be visible in the angle of the anterior chamber. Glaucoma is a common association. The absence of the iris causes marked photophobia, which may be helped by tinted contact lenses.

Ectopia Lentis

Displacement of the lens may occur as an isolated ocular finding. It is due to the weakness of the zonule and can

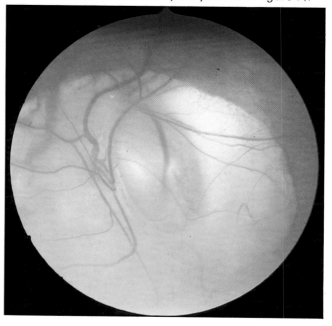

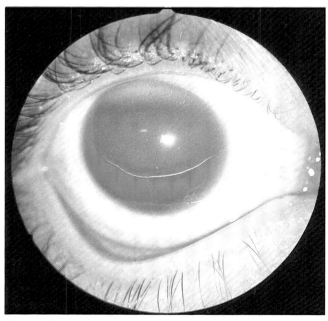

Figure 9. *Aniridia: no iris can be seen; the edge of the lens is visible in the lower third of the red reflex.*

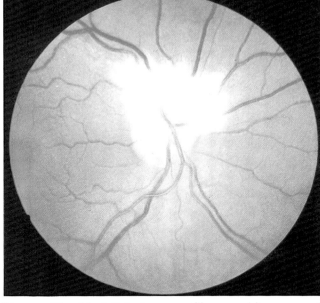

Figure 11. *Medullated nerve fibres: white area of myelinated nerve fibres masking the retinal vessels.*

have a strong hereditary tendency. The edge of the lens may be visible through the pupil (Figure 10).

The condition is also seen as part of Marfan's syndrome, in which there are skeletal abnormalities with elongation of the limbs, particularly the hands and feet

Figure 10. *Ectopia lentis: displacement of the lens upwards and medially.*

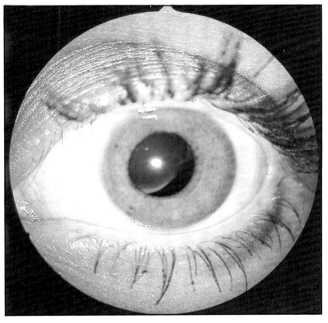

(arachnodactyly). There is generalized muscle wasting and one-third of cases have cardiac lesions which may result in sudden death. Typically the lens is displaced upwards.

Medullated Nerve Fibres

Medullation of the optic nerve usually ceases at the lamina cribrosa. Occasionally, the process extends into the eye to involve nerve fibres in the retina.

The appearance is characteristic (Figure 11). The medullated fibres are white with a feathery edge and the retinal vessels are obscured. The white area is usually continuous with either the upper or lower border of the disc, but occasionally isolated islands may be found away from the optic nerve head.

The visual acuity is not usually affected, but a scotoma corresponding to the lesion may be found on testing the visual field.

Persistent Hyaloid Artery

The hyaloid artery, which forms part of the fetal vascular system to the lens, becomes atrophic in the normal development of the eye. Persistence of all or part of the artery is one of the commoner congenital abnormalities of the eye.

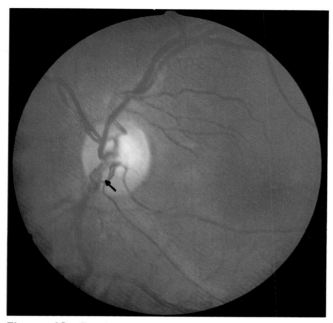

Figure 12. *Persistent hyaloid artery: remnant of the hyaloid artery extending into the vitreous from the centre of the disc.*

The most frequent presentation is a persistent blood vessel or a strand of glial tissue arising from the disc (Figure 12). Occasionally, the remains of the vessel can be found extending forward through the vitreous to its attachment to the back of the lens. The vision is usually unaffected unless the lens is involved.

Retinoblastoma

This rare retinal tumour may be present at birth or may develop shortly afterwards. Its presentation is usually delayed until the tumour is large enough to produce a whitish appearance in the pupil, but earlier diagnosis may be made when a tumour sited on the macula has caused a squint.

The earliest referral is essential as the tumour can spread directly to the brain with fatal consequences. Occasionally, the tumour affects both eyes. A small proportion of cases show a hereditary basis of transmission.

Treatment using a combination of radiotherapy, light coagulation and cryotherapy is possible with small lesions, but usually enucleation is necessary. □

The Eye in Systemic Disease

15

The fundus of the eye offers a unique opportunity for the easy examination of part of the vascular tree and for the early diagnosis of conditions affecting this system.

Arteriosclerosis

The changes of arteriosclerosis appear between the ages of 55 and 60 years and increase with age. These normal ageing changes in the retinal vasculature may at times appear so marked as to look pathological.

The arteries become straightened and the blood column narrows irregularly due to thickening of the inner layers of the arterial wall. As a result of this thickening the reflection of an ophthalmoscope light from the wall of the vessel appears wider and brighter. In the early stages this is described as 'copper wiring', but as the wall becomes more optically dense the description of 'silver wiring' is applied. Eventually the thickening of the wall is so marked that sheathing of the vessel is seen.

At the arteriovenous crossings the vessels share a common adventitia, and the thickening may cause narrowing of the vein which also becomes deflected at a right angle to the artery. The process of arteriosclerosis is often associated with some degree of hypertension, when the fundus appearance is altered by the addition of haemorrhages and exudates.

Hypertension

The appearance of hypertensive retinopathy varies with the age of onset of the disease. In the younger age-group there is widespread narrowing of the arteries due to spasm of the normal vessel walls. When there is co-existing arteriosclerosis the rigidity of some of the vessels results in narrowing of segments of the arteries. Haemorrhages and exudates appear as the hypertension increases in severity.

The haemorrhages are usually flame-shaped as they lie in the superficial nerve fibre layer of the retina, and occur mainly close to the disc. When the haemorrhages are deeply situated in the retina they appear either round or punctate.

The exudates are either 'soft' or 'hard'. The soft exudate caused by infarction of the retina appears as a greyish area and gradually develops into a white spot with a hazy edge. These exudates are widely scattered throughout the retina and vary in size. They tend to disappear when the condition is treated. Hard exudates due to collections of lipids appear as discrete yellowish-white deposits which tend to form at the posterior pole, arranged around the macula in a star-shaped pattern.

Oedema of the retina may be present with mild degrees of hypertension, but it is a marked feature of malignant hypertension (Figures 1 to 3). The appearance of the disc, which becomes hyperaemic and swollen, may be difficult to distinguish from papilloedema due to raised intracranial pressure.

Diabetes

The most important effect of diabetes on the eye is the development of diabetic retinopathy. However, the condition may also affect the lens and extraocular muscles.

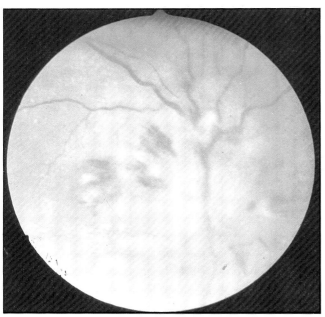

Figure 1. *Malignant hypertension, showing papillo-edema of the disc with flame-shaped haemorrhages, soft exudates (cottonwool spots) and hard exudates.*

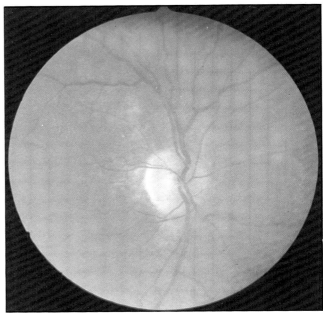

Figure 2. *Malignant hypertension: same case as in Figure 1, three years after treatment with complete resolution of all the signs.*

Lens

A change of refraction towards myopia with blurred distance vision can be a presenting symptom of diabetes, and is caused by the osmotic effect of hyper-

Figure 3. *Malignant hypertension: the hard exudates are arranged around the fovea in a macular star.*

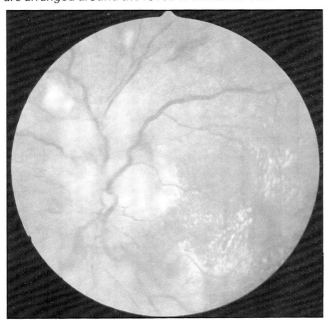

glycaemia. When the diabetes is controlled a further change occurs with the development of hypermetropia. This may be troublesome in the presbyopic age-group who find that they can no longer read small print.

Diabetic patients tend to develop senile cataract at a younger age than nondiabetic patients, but the progression of the lens opacities may be extremely slow. Rapidly developing bilateral cataracts are seen in the uncontrolled juvenile diabetic. Fortunately the condition is uncommon.

Extraocular Muscles

Double vision caused by sudden paralysis of a muscle supplied by the third or sixth cranial nerve can occur with diabetes. Unilateral headache and vomiting may accompany the palsy which usually resolves spontaneously.

Retina

The retinopathy of diabetes is related to the duration rather than the severity of the disease. When the condition has existed for 20 years, 60 per cent of cases will show retinal changes. Evidence seems to suggest that good control will delay the onset of retinopathy but will have little effect on established retinopathy. Diabetic retinopathy is divided into background and proliferative types.

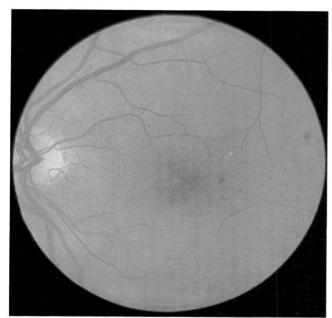

Figure 4. *Background diabetic retinopathy: micro-aneurysms appearing as small red dots.*

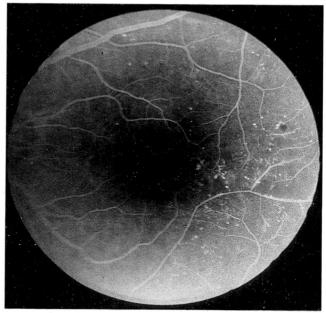

Figure 5. *Fluorescein angiography: same case as in Figure 4, showing extensive vascular changes not visible on routine fundus photography.*

1. Background retinopathy. The earliest sign is venous distension with the formation of aneurysms, which appear as minute red dots scattered over the posterior pole. Small petechial haemorrhages occur as a result of the rupture of these aneurysms (Figure 4). Fluorescein angiography can show these changes which may be overlooked on routine ophthalmoscopic examination (Figure 5).

The haemorrhages may enlarge to form the 'blot' type which usually occur away from the disc, unlike the flame-shaped haemorrhages of arterial disease.

Hard exudates, similar to those seen in hypertension, tend to collect at the posterior pole of the eye. In time, these exudates become absorbed only to reappear elsewhere in the retina (Figure 6). Soft exudates (cotton-wool spots) are less commonly seen.

Background retinopathy does not usually affect the visual acuity unless macular oedema develops. This is characterized by the formation of rings of hard exudates which gradually encroach upon the fovea.

2. Proliferative retinopathy. The ischaemic nature of diabetes may result in neovascularization, although this occurs in only 10 per cent of cases with diabetic retinopathy. It is marked by areas of capillary non-perfusion that can be seen with fluorescein angiography. New vessels develop on the surface of the retina or from the disc (Figure 7) and are liable to rupture if the overlying vitreous contracts, causing severe vitreous

haemorrhage. Organization of this haemorrhage results in the formation of fibrovascular bands (retinitis proliferans) which contract producing further haemorrhage and retinal detachment (Figure 8).

Figure 6. *Background diabetic retinopathy: appearance of exudates and petechial haemorrhages.*

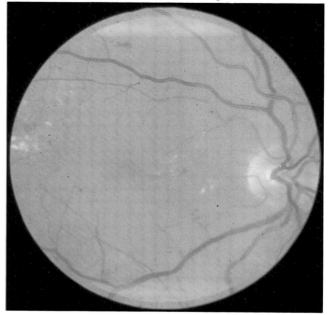

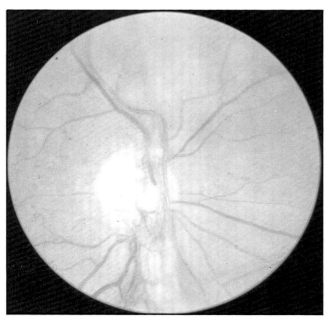

Figure 7. *Proliferative diabetic retinopathy: neovascularization arising from the disc and extending forwards into the vitreous.*

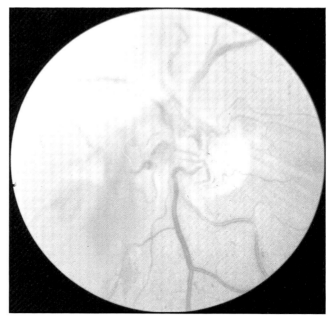

Figure 8. *Proliferative diabetic retinopathy: retinitis proliferans with neovascularization of the disc and a traction detachment of the retina.*

Treatment

Good medical control of diabetes probably helps to delay the onset of retinopathy. Photocoagulation with light or laser beam is now widely used for treatment of

Figure 9. *Photocoagulation, showing discrete white choroidoretinal burns.*

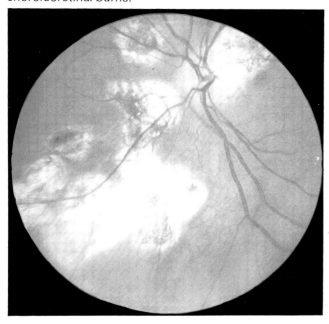

existing retinopathy (Figure 9). This method produces localized burns and is used to treat directly areas of vascular abnormalities that are causing retinal oedema, or to destroy new vessels. Photocoagulation of large areas of the peripheral retina can also be used for neovascularization of the disc. It is thought that destruction of part of the ischaemic retina removes the stimulus for the production of new vessels on the disc.

In advanced diabetic eye disease with fibrovascular proliferations in the vitreous causing retinal detachment, extensive surgery to remove the vitreous (vitrectomy) is required. However, even with the sophisticated instruments now in use, the results of detachment surgery in diabetes are poor.

Thyroid Disease

The term Graves' disease is usually used to describe the combination of hyperthyroidism with eye signs. A small proportion of cases may present with the ocular findings but normal thyroid function tests. The eye signs of Graves' disease are lid retraction, swelling of the lids and conjunctiva, exophthalmos and ophthalmoplegia.

Lid Retraction

In the normal eye the upper lid covers the cornea for about 2 mm and the sclera is not visible above the cornea. Lid retraction occurs in 50 per cent of cases of

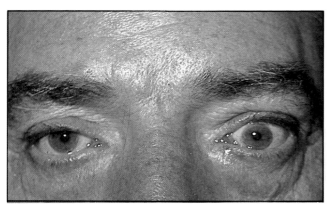

Figure 10. *Thyroid eye disease: retraction of the left upper lid.*

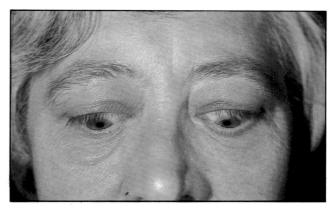

Figure 12. *Thyroid eye disease: lid lag with widening of the gap between the upper lids and the cornea on looking down.*

Graves' disease and although usually bilateral, may be unilateral (Figures 10 and 11). It is possibly due to overaction of the sympathetically supplied levator muscle, although the absence of pupillary dilatation weighs against this theory. An accentuation of the lid retraction occurs when the patient is instructed to look down and the rim of sclera above the cornea becomes wider (lid lag) (Figure 12).

Swelling of the Lids and Conjunctiva

Swelling of the lids may result from the bulging forwards from the overfull orbits, or may be due to oedema. In one-third of cases the conjunctiva is red and swollen (chemosis), particularly over the lateral aspect of the sclera. The patient complains of grittiness and irritation.

Exophthalmos or Proptosis

Exophthalmos is present in up to one-third of cases of Graves' disease and while usually bilateral, may be unilateral. It is marked by retraction of the lower lids with a rim of sclera visible below the cornea (Figure 13).

The protrusion of the eyes is the result of the enlargement of the extraocular muscles and the generalized infiltration of the orbital tissues by mucopolysaccharides and oedema. A cellular infiltration into the muscles gradually develops into a fibrotic process which may result in ophthalmoplegia from muscle paresis.

Ophthalmoplegia

Up to 20 per cent of cases of Graves' disease may suffer from ophthalmoplegia, although many of these may

Figure 11. *Thyroid eye disease: bilateral upper lid retraction but normal relationship of the lower lids to the cornea.*

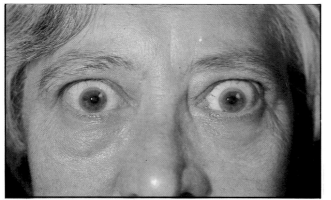

Figure 13. *Thyroid eye disease: bilateral exophthalmos or proptosis shown by retraction of both lower lids.*

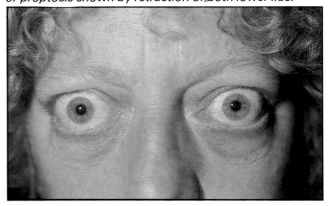

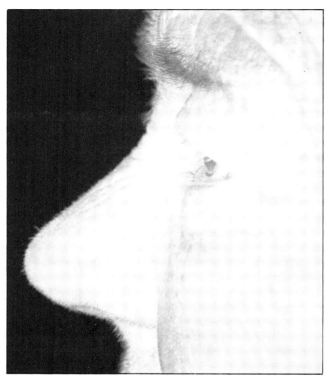

Figure 14. *Myxoedema, showing oedema of the lids with loss of the outer third of the eyebrow.*

have no visual complaints. Double vision, when present, is often worse in the morning. Limited elevation of the eye is the commonest defect occurring as a result of fibrosis and shrinkage of the inferior rectus muscle.

Management

In the mild cases with cosmetically unacceptable lid retraction, guanethidine 5 per cent drops twice daily may be beneficial. However, irritation and redness may occur as a side-effect, together with worsening of the conjunctival chemosis.

Treatment for exposure of the cornea due to inadequate closure of the lids at night should be with lubricant methylcellulose drops by day and chloramphenicol ointment at night.

Ophthalmoplegia is difficult to treat effectively. Occlusion of one eye will avoid the double vision, which may also be lessened by using a prismatic spectacle correction. Surgery to the affected muscles should not be considered until the muscle weakness has been stationary for at least one year, as spontaneous improvement may occur.

Systemic corticosteroids may be indicated when the condition becomes severe. This stage of progressive exophthalmos is marked by failing vision with compression of the optic nerve. The eyes are grossly congested and proptosed and there may be papilloedema and macular oedema. Doses of 120 mg prednisolone daily can be given for three to four days and then reduced. If there is no improvement within a few days surgical decompression to release the intraorbital pressure should be considered.

Myxoedema

Myxoedema is characterized by oedema of the lids, loss of eyelashes and the outer third of the eyebrows (Figure 14). Mild irritation of the eyes may be associated with a diminished tear secretion.

Rheumatoid Arthritis

Ocular involvement in rheumatoid arthritis is not common and is limited to involvement of the tear secretion and the sclera with its overlying episcleral tissue.

Keratoconjunctivitis Sicca

Dryness of the eye due to decreased tear secretion may be accompanied by diminished salivary secretion (Sjögren's syndrome). The eyes are red and sore with occasional sharp pain like that from a foreign body.

Figure 15. *Keratoconjunctivitis sicca: poor tear secretion with excessive mucus production has resulted in strands of mucus adhering to the corneal epithelium (filamentary keratitis).*

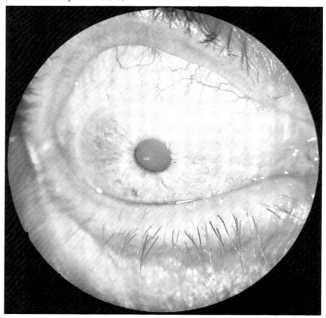

Blinking is painful as the lid crosses the dried cornea. An increased mucus secretion results in strands of mucus adhering to the corneal epithelium (filamentary keratitis) (Figure 15). A tear secretion test (Schirmer's test), with strips of filter paper placed in the conjunctival sac, can be used.

Treatment by replacement or artificial tears is with methylcellulose drops. If there is excessive mucus secretion, acetylcysteine drops 5 per cent—a mucolytic agent—can be used.

Episcleral and Scleral Changes

A nodular episcleritis with a localized raised red area can cause some pain (Figure 16). The lesion usually resolves spontaneously over a period of weeks and leaves no permanent damage. Local corticosteroid drops will usually hasten this natural remission.

Scleritis is a far more serious complication of ocular rheumatoid arthritis. The inflammation may be either diffuse or localized, but it is always painful (Figure 17). Treatment with systemic corticosteroids may be indicated, especially if perforation of the globe threatens.

Sarcoidosis

Thirty per cent of patients with sarcoidosis have ocular involvement. Uveitis has already been discussed on page 45. Lacrimal gland involvement may result in severe

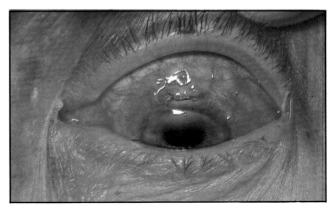

Figure 17. *Scleritis in rheumatoid arthritis: localized area of inflammation with necrosis of the sclera.*

keratoconjunctivitis sicca. Simultaneous enlargement of the salivary glands is known as Mikulicz's syndrome (Figure 18).

Angioid Streaks

This uncommon degenerative change is of interest because of its association with a number of other systemic conditions in which there is degeneration of elastic tissue, i.e. pseudoxanthoma elasticum, Paget's disease and sickle cell disease.

The fundus changes are characteristic. A network of

Figure 16. *Episcleritis in rheumatoid arthritis: localized nodular area of inflammation.*

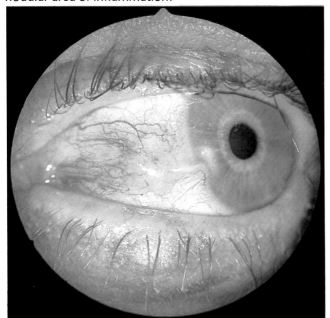

Figure 18. *Sarcoidosis: bilateral enlargement of the parotid glands.*

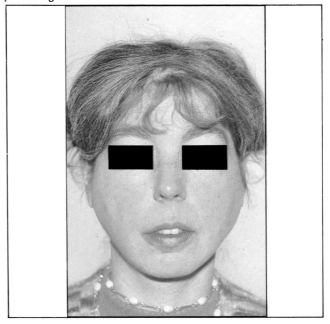

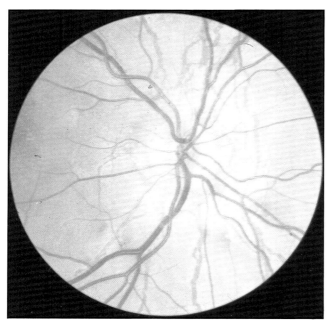

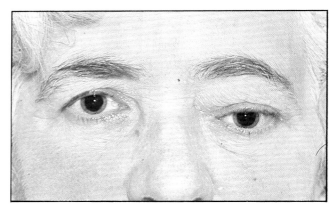

Figure 21. *Frontal mucocele, causing downward displacement of the left eye and double vision.*

Figure 19. *Angioid streaks: appearance of the lesions around the disc; sometimes associated with pseudoxanthoma elasticum, Paget's disease and sickle cell anaemia.*

reddish-brown spokes radiates from a ring of similar colour which circles the disc (Figure 19). Eyes with angioid streaks are especially vulnerable to trauma and have been called 'eggshell' eyes.

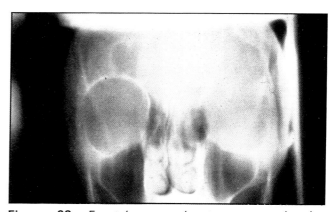

Figure 20. *Metastatic tumour: secondary deposit in the choroid from carcinoma of the breast.*

Figure 22. *Frontal mucocele: tomogram showing erosion of the roof of the left orbit.*

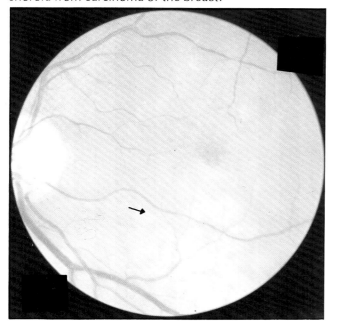

Metastatic Tumours

The eye is sometimes the site of blood-borne metastases. The tumour emboli are usually found at the posterior pole. The appearance is distinctive with a flat, mottled grey lesion with ill-defined edges (Figure 20).

The commonest primary growth is carcinoma of the breast with the lungs and thyroid occasionally implicated.

Nasopharyngeal Disease

Spread of infection from the sinuses can cause orbital cellulitis, while infiltrating pharyngeal carcinoma and frontal mucocele may be a cause of unilateral proptosis or displacement of the globe (Figures 21 and 22).

Many conditions involving the central nervous system affect the eye. The ocular symptoms may be obvious, as with visual loss or double vision. Occasionally, however, the symptoms may be slight and only careful investigation will reveal unsuspected signs that can help to localize the possible site of the lesion.

Tests of Visual Function

Visual Acuity

Accurate assessment of the visual acuity is necessary to distinguish those cases of papilloedema due to raised intracranial pressure with normal vision from papillitis with a swollen optic disc but reduced vision.

Distance and near vision should be tested with glasses if necessary. The common practice of assessing only the near vision is inadequate as a normal level (N.5) for near vision can be achieved when the distance vision is reduced to 6/12.

Visual Fields

Both central and peripheral visual fields must be charted. Central fields assessed with a Bjerrum screen are accurate only from the central fixation spot out to 30 degrees, beyond which a perimeter must be used (see page 13).

The confrontation method can be used to elicit gross field defects but cannot be relied upon to detect small areas of blindness. Certain visual field defects may indicate very accurately sites of interruption of the visual pathway, while others are nonspecific. Figure 1 shows the three main parts of the visual pathway, lesions of which produce characteristic field defects.

1. Anterior to the optic chiasma. The unilateral field loss may involve part or all of the field of vision. The eye must be examined to eliminate any ocular causes for field defects, such as senile macular degeneration producing a central scotoma similar to that of retrobulbar neuritis.

2. Optic chiasma. The typical bitemporal hemianopia of a pituitary tumour is caused by pressure on the crossing nasal fibres. Pressure on other parts of the optic chiasma by a meningioma or aneurysm may produce different field defects. However, they usually have some bitemporal defect although the loss may be small and easily overlooked.

3. Posterior to the optic chiasma. The field defects are homonymous with a right-sided lesion causing loss of the opposite side (left) of each visual field. If half the field is affected a hemianopia is present, while the term quadrantanopia is used when only a small segment is involved.

Lesions of the optic tract tend to be incongruous (dissimilar in shape), as the fibres from corresponding retinal areas do not lie together. Temporal lobe lesions cause an upper quadrantanopia while those in the parietal lobe tend to produce a lower quadrantanopia. Lesions affecting the more posterior part of the optic radiations tend to produce field defects that are congruous (similar in shape) with the central macular field unaffected.

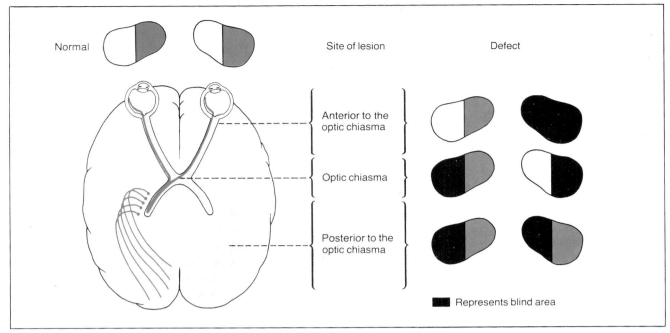

Figure 1. *Visual field defects.*

Colour Vision

Defective colour vision is common with both retinal and optic nerve disorders. Red/green discrimination can be tested with Ishihara plates for the early diagnosis of toxic and retrobulbar neuritis.

Examination of the Pupils

Routine examination of the pupils is often cursory and the information gained of little diagnostic value. A properly performed examination may obviate unnecessary investigations in some cases and may be life-saving for the unconscious patient.

Normal Pupil Reactions

1. Direct light response—constriction of the pupil with direct light.

2. Consensual light response—simultaneous constriction of the opposite pupil.

3. Near response—simultaneous and equal constriction of both pupils when accommodating and converging the eyes.

The size of the normal pupil is achieved by a balance between the constrictor muscle fibres supplied by the parasympathetic nervous system and the dilator muscle fibres controlled by the sympathetic system. A difference in size of 1 mm between the two pupils may be regarded as normal as long as the pupil reactions are normal. In early childhood and over the age of 60 the pupils tend to be small and dilate poorly with mydriatic drops. The pupils are larger in adolescence and when myopia is present.

The Abnormal Pupil

Large Pupil

A large pupil may be caused by:

1. Mydriatic drops instilled by the patient or a previous examiner.

2. Optic neuritis involving the afferent pathway of the pupillary reflex, so that the pupil on the affected side is slightly larger.

3. Third cranial nerve palsy, especially when due to nerve compression by aneurysms or tumour. Vascular infarction of the third nerve as occurs in diabetes tends to spare the pupil because of the double blood supply to the oculomotor and pupilloconstrictor fibres.

4. Adie's syndrome occurring in women aged 20 to 30, in which the dilated pupil does not react to light but constricts slowly with convergence. The pupil also constricts with 2.5 per cent methacholine, which has no effect on the normal pupil. The condition, thought to be due to degeneration in the ciliary ganglion, is associated with loss of tendon reflexes.

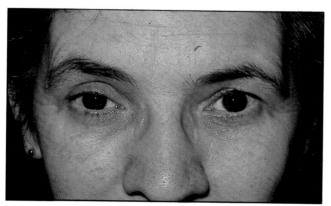

Figure 2. *Horner's syndrome: ptosis, miosis and anhydrosis due to interruption of the sympathetic nerve supply.*

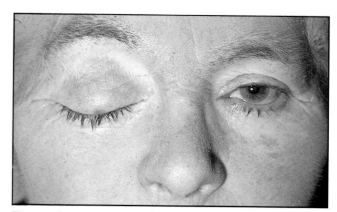

Figure 3. *Ptosis: paralysis of levator palpebral muscle supplied by third cranial nerve, due to intracranial tumour.*

5. Injury, in which the constrictor muscle fibres are torn resulting in traumatic mydriasis.

Small Pupil

A small pupil may be caused by:

1. Miotic drops for glaucoma.

2. Horner's syndrome due to damage to the sympathetic nerve supply to the pupil. The miosis of the pupil is accompanied by a ptosis of the lid and anhydrosis (loss of sweating) on the same side of the face. Interruption of the long course of the sympathetic supply can occur in the brainstem due to posterior inferior cerebellar artery occlusion, or in the cervical cord as a result of syringomyelia. Apical bronchial carcinoma (Pancoast tumour), tumours of the thyroid, larynx and oesophagus, and carotid arteriography are among the commoner lesions in the neck (Figure 2).

3. Argyll–Robertson pupil, usually associated with neurosyphilis, is occasionally found in patients with diabetes and multiple sclerosis. The small unequal pupils do not react to light but react with accommodation. There is no dilatation with atropine.

The Pupils in the Unconscious Patient

The state of the pupils is one of the most important investigations in the unconscious patient. The findings must be considered together with details of possible head injury, metabolic coma or drug intoxication.

Unilateral dilatation of the pupil suggests 'coning' due to prolapse of the temporal lobe through the tentorium requiring immediate action. Untreated, this will develop into bilateral dilatation of the pupils with no reaction to light. Both pupils may be involved in cases of severe brain damage, epilepsy and drug overdose. Bilateral constriction of the pupils may occur with pontine haemorrhage and opiate poisoning.

Extraocular Muscle Function

The presentation of ocular palsy has already been mentioned on page 92.

Ocular Palsy

The third cranial nerve supplies the superior, medial and inferior rectus muscles and the inferior oblique muscle. It also supplies the levator palpebrae muscle and the constrictor fibres of the pupil. A complete palsy of this nerve produces ptosis and loss of adduction, elevation and depression, with dilatation of the pupil (Figures 3 to 6). Pain associated with third nerve palsy is usually due to aneurysm.

Figure 4. *Right third cranial nerve palsy: loss of adduction.*

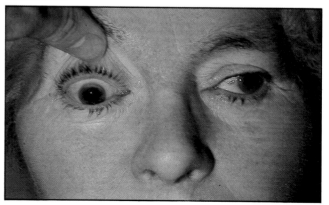

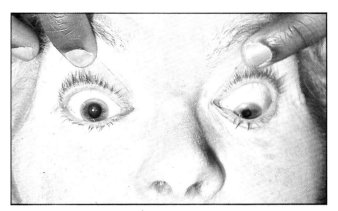

Figure 5. *Right third cranial nerve palsy: loss of depression with dilated pupil.*

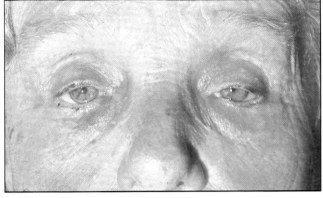

Figure 7. *Senile ptosis.*

The fourth cranial nerve supplies the superior oblique muscle. Despite its long intracranial course, fourth nerve palsy is uncommon and when present is usually the result of trauma.

The sixth cranial nerve supplies the lateral rectus muscle, palsy of which results in loss of abduction.

Bilateral Ptosis

Bilateral ptosis may be present as part of an ageing change (involutionary or senile ptosis, Figure 7) or may be part of a general condition.

In myasthenia gravis, bilateral ptosis is nearly always a feature and may be the only sign of the condition (Figure 8). Diplopia due to muscle involvement may be either horizontal or vertical (Figures 9 and 10). The symptoms may be intermittent at first, but are usually worse towards evening when the muscle fatigue is most marked. Weakness of the facial muscles tends to give a somewhat expressionless myasthenic facies. The diag-

nosis can be confirmed with the Tensilon test, using intravenous edrophonium chloride, when an improvement in muscle power becomes obvious.

Myotonia dystrophica is a rare cause of bilateral ptosis (Figure 11). There is an associated myotonia, wasting of facial muscles, frontal baldness and testicular atrophy with posterior subcapsular cataracts.

Bilateral ptosis is also seen in the rare group of ocular

Figure 8. *Myasthenia gravis: bilateral ptosis of myasthenic facies.*

Figure 6. *Right sixth cranial nerve palsy: loss of abduction.*

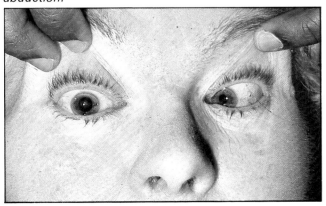

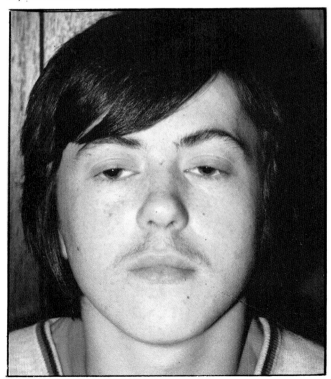

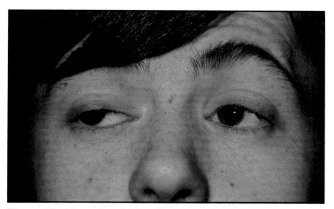

Figure 9. *Myasthenia gravis: weakness of adduction.*

and parietal lobe lesions produce different responses. It can also be used to differentiate vascular and neoplastic lesions (which may give different responses) and to measure visual acuity in children.

Pendular nystagmus is usually the result of poor vision present from birth. Albinism and congenital cataract are two of the many causes. Jerk nystagmus is caused by a neurological lesion, involving either the vestibular system, the cerebellum or the brain stem.

myopathies in which the eye muscles are involved by a dystrophy, which occasionally involves muscles of the face, pharynx and upper limbs (Figures 12 and 13).

Nystagmus

This is a rhythmical involuntary oscillation of both eyes. It may be horizontal, vertical or rotatory in direction. There are two main types: 'pendular' nystagmus, in which the movement in each direction is of equal speed, and 'jerk' nystagmus when one movement is fast and the other slow. It can occur normally at the extreme positions of gaze (end-point nystagmus) and can be induced in the normal patient by his viewing a rotating drum painted with black and white stripes (opticokinetic nystagmus), when the eye movements are similar to those produced when looking out of a moving train.

The opticokinetic response can be used to differentiate the site of postchiasmal lesions, since temporal

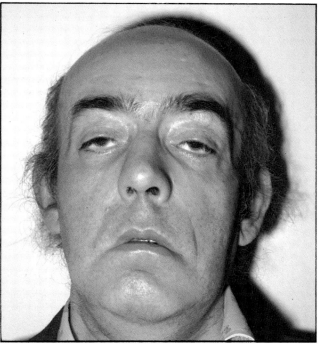

Figure 11. *Myotonia dystrophica: bilateral ptosis, wasting of facial muscles and frontal balding.*

Figure 10. *Myasthenia gravis: weakness of abduction.*

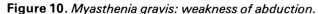
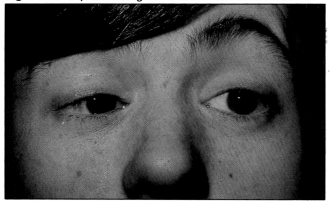

Figure 12. *Ocular myopathy: bilateral ptosis.*

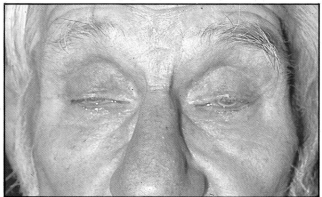

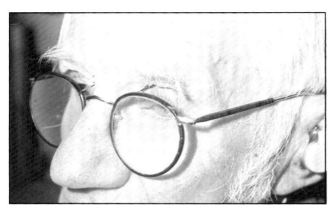

Figure 13. *Ocular myopathy: correction of ptosis with 'ptosis props' attached to the spectacle frame.*

Examination of the Disc

The normal appearance of the disc has been discussed on page 51. The two important pathological changes in the disc are oedema and optic atrophy.

Oedema

The term papilloedema is used to describe swelling of the disc that is noninflammatory in origin. The term papillitis describes swelling of the disc that occurs with optic neuritis. The appearance of papilloedema and papillitis are identical, but the differentiation is made by the reduction in visual acuity that occurs with papillitis.

Papilloedema is nearly always bilateral. The early case is marked by blurring of the disc margins (Figure 14). As the swelling progresses the physiological pit may be lost, but this depends on its original size. If the diagnosis of papilloedema is in doubt, fluorescein angiography will show a characteristic leakage of dye from the dilated disc capillaries (Figure 15). The disc may become hyperaemic and the veins are engorged. In later stages oedema spreads from the disc to the surrounding retina. Flame-shaped haemorrhages and exudates are seen on or near the disc margin (Figure 16). In chronic papilloedema the disc becomes pale due to gliosis (Figure 17). The swelling gradually subsides until the final stage of optic atrophy is reached (Figure 18).

Papilloedema is most commonly associated with raised intracranial pressure caused by cerebral tumours. It is also seen with malignant hypertension. The vision is usually normal unless the macula is involved by exudates, but the blind spot is enlarged.

In contrast to the slow loss of vision with papilloedema, the vision deteriorates rapidly with optic neuritis. When the condition is unilateral it is usually due to multiple sclerosis. It occurs mainly between the ages of 20 and 45 years and is rarely seen after the age of 60. There is a sudden onset of pain in the eye, which is worse on movement. Loss of central vision occurs

Figure 14. *Papilloedema: early case with blurred disc margin, hyperaemia and venous engorgement.*

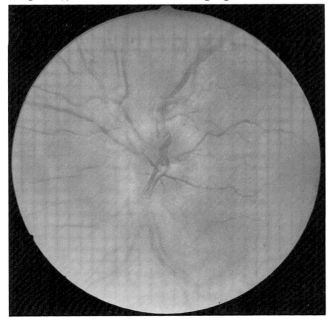

Figure 15. *Papilloedema: leakage of fluorescein dye around the disc.*

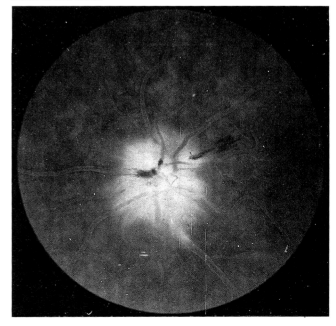

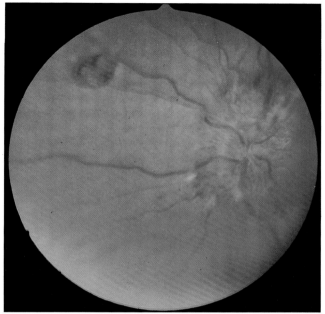

Figure 16. *Papilloedema: late case with flame-shaped haemorrhages and exudates.*

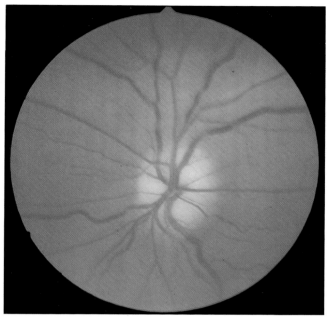

Figure 18. *Papilloedema: late stage with swelling of the disc being replaced by the pallor of optic atrophy.*

Figure 17. *Chronic papilloedema: gliosis of the disc causes pallor and masking of the vessels.*

Figure 19. *Optic atrophy: comparison between the normal pink disc and the white atrophic disc.*

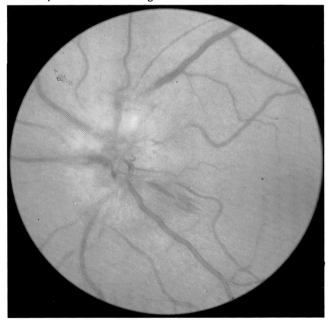

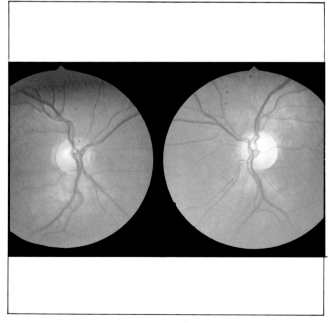

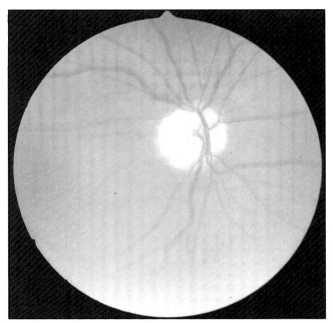

Figure 20. *Optic atrophy: pearly white disc with sharp margins (primary optic atrophy).*

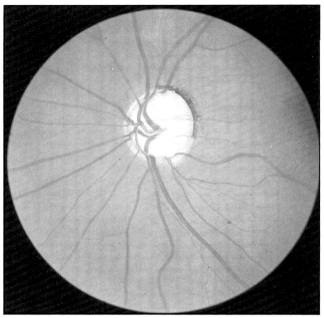

Figure 21. *Glaucomatous optic atrophy: cupping of the disc with displacement of the vessels.*

within several days and varies from a slight deficit to a dense central scotoma. Vision is often made worse by a hot bath or exercise. The pupil on the affected side may be slightly dilated and reacts poorly to direct light (afferent pupil defect). The disc is swollen when the demyelination involves the anterior portion of the optic nerve. The term retrobulbar neuritis is used to describe a lesion affecting the trunk of the optic nerve when no ophthalmoscopic changes are seen.

A variable recovery of vision occurs over several weeks, but there may be recurrences. The general prognosis of the condition is uncertain, but other signs of multiple sclerosis may not become manifest for many years.

Optic Atrophy

Atrophy of the fibres of the optic nerve is characterized by impairment of visual function and pallor of the optic disc (Figure 19).

The normal disc is paler on the temporal than the nasal side, and is paler in babies. The appearance of the atrophic disc varies with the cause of the atrophy. When there has been no previous oedema of the disc, it is pearly white with a sharp margin (primary optic atrophy; Figure 20), and the vessels can be seen to pass from the retina across the surface of the disc. This is in contrast to the greyish-white appearance of the disc after papilloedema, the gliosis tending to mask the vessels and blur the disc margin (secondary optic atrophy).

In glaucomatous optic atrophy there is loss of tissue of the optic disc so that the vessels tend to disappear over the edge of the enlarged physiological cup (Figure 21).

The fibres of the optic nerve run from the retinal ganglion cells to the lateral geniculate body and interruption at any point along this pathway will produce optic atrophy.   ☐

Ocular Pharmacology

Topical application of drugs is effective for most conditions involving the anterior segment of the eye. Systemic administration and local injections into the subconjunctival or retrobulbar space are necessary to achieve therapeutic levels for the retina and choroid. A list of commonly used drugs is given in Table 1. Drops are usually more easily applied by the patient and avoid the blurred vision caused by the smearing of the cornea with ointments. The use of methylcellulose, as in Isopto Carpine, and polyvinyl alcohol, as in Sno Pilo, increase the viscosity of the solutions, which is said to increase the contact time of the solutions with the eye and is more comfortable for the patient.

Anti-infective Preparations

Antibacterial

Topical chloramphenicol is the drug of choice. It has a wide spectrum of antibacterial activity and rarely gives rise to allergic reactions. 0.5 per cent drops should be used not less than four times each day in acute bacterial conjunctivitis, and the dosage may be more frequent during the first 48 hours of use. One per cent ointment is applied at night to maintain treatment while the eyes are shut.

Neomycin also has a wide spectrum of activity, but due to allergic skin reactions and its toxic effect on the corneal epithelium it should be used with caution.

Gentamicin, tetracyclines and sulphacetamide may also be used topically.

Antiviral

Idoxuridine is effective against herpes simplex virus, but prolonged use can cause toxicity with damage to the corneal epithelium, redness and watering of the eye. It should be given in 0.5 per cent ointment five times daily. 0.1 per cent drops are also available.

Vidarabine and trifluorothymidine are recent alternative forms of treatment. All antiviral therapy should be supervised by an ophthalmic department.

Anti-inflammatory Preparations

Corticosteroid preparations are invaluable but potentially dangerous drugs. Their combination with antibiotics does nothing to lessen this risk. Indiscriminate use can result in viral and fungal infection, steroid-induced glaucoma and cataract.

Topical prednisolone, betamethasone and dexamethasone are effective against inflammation in the anterior part of the eye, but systemic therapy is necessary for the posterior eye.

Oxyphenbutazone is a non-corticosteroid preparation used in ointment form. It is not as active against inflammation as the corticosteroids but it does not produce the same complications.

Sodium cromoglycate is a recent addition to the antiallergic drugs and can be used for hayfever, conjunctivitis and vernal catarrh.

Numerous antihistamine and decongestant preparations are available for the mildly irritable eye.

Preparations for Glaucoma

The intraocular pressure is maintained by a balance between the production and drainage of aqueous humour from the eye, and treatment of glaucoma is aimed at these two sites.

Miotics which constrict the pupil also increase the outflow of aqueous humour. Pilocarpine drops 1 to 4 per cent are most commonly used.

Adrenaline and guanethidine drops may be used in open-angle glaucoma, but because of the dilating effect on the pupil, they should not be given if the anterior chamber is shallow.

Timolol, used as drops to increase aqueous humour outflow, is a successful new drug, although adequate control of pressure over a long period has yet to be proved.

Aqueous humour production is reduced by the carbonic anhydrase inhibitors acetazolamide and dichlorphenamide, which may be given systemically in conjunction with local therapy.

Table 1. Commonly used drugs.

	Chemical Name	Proprietary Name
Anti-infective		
Antibacterial	Chloramphenicol	Minims, Chloromycetin
	Gentamicin	Genticin
	Neomycin	Minims, Myciguent, Nivemycin
	Tetracyclines	Achromycin, Aureomycin
	Sulphacetamide	Albucid, Isopto Cetamide, Minims, Ocusol
Antiviral	Idoxuridine	Dendrid, Idoxene, Kerecid, Ophthalmadine
	Vidarabine	Vira-A
	Trifluorothymidine	Viroptic
Anti-inflammatory		
Corticosteroids	Hydrocortisone	Hydrocortistab
	Prednisolone	Predsol
	Betamethasone	Betnesol
	Dexamethasone	Maxidex
Non-corticosteroids	Oxyphenbutazone	Tanderil
	Sodium cromoglycate	Opticrom
Antihistamine and decongestant	Xylometazoline, antazoline and naphazoline, zinc sulphate	Otrivine-Antistin, Vasocon-A, Zincfrin
Glaucoma	Pilocarpine	Isopto Carpine, Minims, Sno Pilo
	Adrenaline	Eppy, Isopto Epinal, Simplene
	Guanethidine	Ganda
	Timolol maleate	Timoptol
	Acetazolamide	Diamox
	Dichlorphenamide	Daranide, Oratrol
Mydriatics	Tropicamide	Mydriacyl
	Cyclopentolate	Mydrilate
	Homatropine	Minims
	Atropine	Isopto atropine, Minims, Opulets
Anaesthesia	Oxybuprocaine	Minims
	Proxymetacaine	Ophthaine
	Lignocaine	Xylocaine
	Amethocaine	Minims
Artificial tears	Hypromellose	Isopto, Tears Naturale

Mydriatics

Dilatation of the pupil may be necessary for diagnostic reasons, e.g. to examine the fundus, or for treatment, e.g. to limit pupillary spasm and the formation of posterior synechiae in uveitis.

Diagnostic Mydriasis

0.5 per cent tropicamide achieves adequate rapid dilatation without blurring of vision. This makes it the ideal mydriatic for routine examination of the fundus.

10 per cent phenylephrine may be used to dilate the constricted pupils in the patient with chronic simple glaucoma on miotic therapy.

1 per cent atropine ointment is used to achieve adequate mydriasis with complete cycloplegia before routine refraction in children. Ointment is preferable to drops which may produce toxic reactions due to excess absorption.

Therapeutic Mydriasis

The choice of drugs depends on the duration of mydriasis required. Cyclopentolate and homatropine are active for one to two days while atropine lasts for seven to ten days.

Local Anaesthesia

Oxybuprocaine or proxymetacaine are short-acting anaesthetics used for examination of the eye or the removal of small foreign bodies.

Amethocaine with its longer action is used for minor surgical procedures. The eye should be padded after using amethocaine in order to protect the anaesthetized cornea against air-borne foreign bodies.

Local anaesthetic drugs should not be given to relieve pain as their continued use may damage the corneal epithelium.

Artificial Tears

Hypromellose (hydroxypropyl methylcellulose) is available in various strengths for tear replacement. The drops should be taken as often as necessary to relieve discomfort.

Index